A Path to Relapse Prevention

Book by the Author

The Other Door, Poetic Exhortations, 1980
The Tale of Willie the Humpback Whale, 1981
Two Modern Short Stories of Immigrant Life, 1984
The Safe Child/The Unsafe Child, 1985

◊

The Last Trumpet and the Woodbridge Demon
Angelic Renegades & Rephaim Giants

◊

Tiamat, Mother of Demon I
Gwyllion, Daughter of the Tiamat II
Revenge of the Tiamat III

◊

Mantic ore: Day of the Beast

Everyday's an Adventure
[Short Stories]

Chasing the Sun
[Travels of D.L Siluk]

Islam, In Search of Satan's Rib

The Rape of Angelina of Glastonbury 1099 AD
[The Green Knight]

A Path to Sobriety,
The Inside Passage
Volume I

A Path to Relapse Prevention,
The Inside Passage
Volume II

Aftercare, a Path through It
The Inside Passage
Volume III

Romancing San Francisco
[Volume I]

A Romance in Augsburg
[Volume II]

Where the Birds Don't Sing
[Volume III]

Death on Demand
[Seven Suspenseful Short Stories]

Death by Desire
[Nine Stores of Suspense]
[To be released]

The Mumbler,
Slayer by the Second Self
[To be released]

The Curse of the Viper Family
[The Abyss Virus Worm]
[To be released]

The Fruit Cake
[A Comedy-Tragedy]
[To be released]

*

A Path to Relapse Prevention

✦

The Inside Passage
Volume II

----A Common Sense Book----
On Understanding the Sensitively, Thinking
And Repair work needed for the Alcoholic and Drug Inflicted

Dennis L. Siluk

iUniverse, Inc.
New York Lincoln Shanghai

A Path to Relapse Prevention
The Inside Passage Volume II

iUniverse, Inc.

For information address:
iUniverse
2021 Pine Lake Road, Suite 100
Lincoln, NE 68512
www.iuniverse.com

ISBN: 0-595-29391-3

Printed in the United States of America

<u>Dedicated to:</u>

…All the hardheads out there
Trying to sober up…don't stop,
Stay sober…and drug free,
Life is short enough…

◊

Love and Butterflies

[For Elsie Siluk, my mother]

She fought a good battle,
The last of many—
Until there was nothing left;—
Where at once was plenty.

And so, poised and dignified—
She said, farewell in her own way;—
And left behind,
A grand old time,
Room for another:—
Love and Butterflies…
That was my mother.

Dlsiluk 7/03

Contents

Part One

Prelude: The Inside Passage 3

CHAPTER 1   Introduction on Understanding Prevention 5
      [Plus 'The Calling,' and 'Rosa's Story,' from Peru]

CHAPTER 2   Similarities: Sex Addiction vs. Alcoholism [part I]........10

CHAPTER 3   Similarities: Gambling vs. Alcoholic behavior [part II]...13

CHAPTER 4   Behavioral Stages of Alcoholism 16

CHAPTER 5   Discussion on Behavior: Trust 19

CHAPTER 6   Discussion on Behavior: Criticism 22

CHAPTER 7   Discussion on Behavior: Triggers for Relapse 24

CHAPTER 8   Discussion on Behavior: Self-Esteem 26

CHAPTER 9   Resistance and Co-dependency 30

CHAPTER 10 A Look at some Characteristics of ACA's....................33

CHAPTER 11 Prevention: My Philosophy Statement........................35

CHAPTER 12 Prevention Zones and the Secret 38

CHAPTER 13 Lifestyle choices and the 12-steps 43
      [a review]

CHAPTER 14 Drugs and Poisons 48
      [a birds eye view]

Notes 51

    1-on Confusion and Thinking
    2-on Living on the streets
    3-on Books on the subject
    4-on Recovery and Limitations
    5-on Graphs

The Lonely Child 53

    [A commentary on the needs of a child, a story on love]

Part Two

The Story : "A Woman in Pain" 57

Captions of Other Books by the Author 79

Acknowledgements

Thanks go to:

Dr. Patricia J. Sullwold, VA MED Ctr. for
Keeping me alive these past 15-years;
My wife Rosa for her ongoing
Support in my writings and devotion,
And my mother Elsie Siluk for her help
During my early recovery period
[Who has recently passed on to meet her Maker]

+

"Nothing is free; your bazaar alcoholism or drug induced behavior may reap its rewards now—but later on the tab must be paid."

Dlsiluk

PART ONE

Prelude

◆

[The Inside Passage]

Before we get into the bulk of book let me try and capture just one impression, if you do not mind. In prevention one must repeat to oneself the word 'balance,' so as not to forget it;—you will see this word here and there within the book. This word, both—counselor and client, must remember, the reason being, one-size does not fit all in this recovery-prevention hypothesis.

Your program can be different than your neighbor's,—different than the other person's—why? Ask the question, "Why not?" Because you are different, your personality, your emotional make up, your creativity, your character, your spiritual beliefs, culture, psychosocial background, your private life, your gender, your occupation, they all play a part in making you just a little different than the next human being. All-in-all, what we see here then, is really a different 'anyone,' and this 'anyone, or someone, or everyone' have/has different needs, wants, goals,—and this 'someone', like it or not, is you, yes, Y.O.U! All such things must be brought into the picture. Again one-size does not fit all in the world of recovery, and prevention.

During times of what I call, high-tide [rough times that is], balance in a person's life is hard to hang on to. An example might be, 'stress'. If you sense a trigger nearby [coming], or you are being triggered because of stress, move on over, let go of it, whatever you are hanging on to, that is. And that might be to stop involvement with those who are not good for your sobriety. Ask yourself the question, "Why should I stick around here…around someone who is negative all the time?" They bring you down, make you uneasy, move on over, let them have your chair,—forever. Find people who do not irritate you, appreciate you. No need to explain this to anyone, just do it, they will find someone else to play god with. This is your sobriety, your time, and your equilibrium; this also goes for jobs, court time, anything that involves stress. As one acquires more sobriety time, than you can take on more; also,—this is the time to learn how to differentiate between feelings and thinking, or better put, emotions vs. thoughts, s/he will be building up more tolerance for battles in the future. But you can't expect a newborn to go out and fight the world. The recovering person has to know his/her levels of tolerance, and stay within them.

Let me give you an example. I had about two years of sobriety at the time, and I just gone through a divorce. I put $300 down to rent an apartment, and the next day my mother said, "Why not live with me for a year, save your money, and you can maybe buy a house," something like that. And so I said, 'ok,' it sounded great.

Now I had given the landlord a check, so I could stop it, and so, when I called him, he said "No, you cannot have the money back, and if you stop the check, you are responsible for six months rent, but I'll overlook that if you leave the check alone." Well I thought and thought and thought on this. Now alcoholics respond on emotions more than thinking [usually], and I was angry, and wanted to show him, not sure what I wanted to show him, but something, possible he could not get away with this legal thing, even though it was legal—it doesn't make sense, right? I know, but that's just how we think; any how, I was going to stop payment on the check, and then I got thinking. First, I did sign a contract, second, I was responsible for it, third, I'd get $300 back within the first month of living with my mother, whom was charging me only $100 to live at her place. Forth, I would not have to go to court, fight this person, who was right in principle, yet I felt since only 24-hours had elapsed, I should get my money back; well, I left it alone. And once I let go of it, I slept well, and right or wrong, I did not have to go through the stress. I lost $300, but kept good credit with other people, no court, and got my money back in 60-days besides; you can't beat them odds.

So we got to balance our do's and don't out. OK? Ok. You pick the battles, not your neighbor who will say, "Get him, and get him good, how he dare do this to you..." and then he runs off to some unknown hiding place, saying, "That's my advice." Yes they get you all riled up and leave you out for the crows. Plus they do not know your condition, only their cheap advice. Free advice is normally, what it sounds like, low-browed at best. Find a real friend, one that will give you time, and be there for you. Look at all the corners, then make a decision.

1

Introduction on Understanding Prevention

To understand, or even work with the concept of Prevention, it is worthwhile for the person involved, to investigate its nature and its secret; for it has both. And in the following pages, I will try to unveil just that. No more, no less. We are going to look at an assortment of things, elements if you will. And at the end of this book, if you make it that far, if you make it through the book that is, there will be my Philosophy Statement on Prevention, to review if you wish. I put it at the end of the book simply because I do not want anyone to get confused with the forthcoming chapters; by and large, it leads up to it anyway, I felt it simply blends better this way.

Those people who are dealing with Alcoholism, for the most part, I am most directing this book to, but don't put it down, if you've read my first book on addiction, you will understand why. We will look at the whole addiction arena; from gambling to sex and drugs per se. [Drugs are packaged in with alcoholism.] To the non-addicted, this will be quite informative.

□

When I think about this book I think about the poem Robert Frost wrote called, "The Mending Wall," I was going to make it a subtitle to the book, but decided against it, yet I want to look at how I see the poem with how I see prevention.

First, it is not how we deal with addiction per se, for although that is the dilemma we face here, it is not where the roots are, it is rather the surface, and we need to get underneath it, or put another way, underground, that is where the problem that bothers me is, which is coping with sobriety. Yes, right where the roots get the nourishment. Second, when I say "Mending Wall," I am referring to the protagonist, you, the abuser, the user, the dependent, and possible you the tag along [co-dependent]. But what am I really saying? Well, it is just this:—we addicted people build walls around ourselves. We wall ourselves in, oh yes we do, believe it or not—I know someone out there is saying, 'hogwash'. If that is not obvious, you are still walled in my friend. Having said that, let's go to another level.

I want to back track a little, and then get back to where we where headed. This being my second book on 'addictions' I wrote, and my 20th book in publication to date, I want to let you know I have 17-years working in the addiction field, so you're not getting a recruit, second, I have worked in the behavior science field 30-years; and last but not lest I have over 19-years sobriety. Whenever you talk or read, or watch anything in the addiction field, be it alcoholism, drugs, compulsive gambling, eating disorders, sex, know who you are talking to, or reading. As I used to tell my clients, look for the credentials, if there are none go find someone who has them. Plus every counselor is not made for every client. And last but not least, my philosophy, as I explained in my first book on addiction, "A Path to Sobriety," is, and remains so in this book, "To use whatever resources work for you, to remain sober." Let me add, in working with a number of different clients with dual disorders, I find: *nobody really cares what you know until you show how much you care.* I will try to be sensitive as well as putting as little humor in my books as is in my soul to do so, that is, make it an enjoyable to read,—without destroying the seriousness of the material.

I find we recovering people have had enough pain;—we really do not need anymore, we've lost, and lost and lost, I will try my best to make you a winner in this book, but you got to accept it. However if I fail in this, it is either you or me that need to get additional counseling, if it is me, I will seek it.

Having said all that, let me also add, I do not get into the god thing all that much, but I will have you know, without God, we [or I] are but fragmented pieces of a puzzle trying to be put back together again. I have found in this field that God is most gracious, if you try, He will help, even if you deny Him. And when you go to AA, NA or GA, or for that matter, any emotional, or helping group, to include the 12 or 16 step groups, God plays a part. We can choose our higher power, in any manner we wish, but make it higher than you, that is the trick. In essence what the counselor is saying or AA is preaching, is that, you need someone bigger than you. You've tried it alone, and it doesn't work. You need humanity. Get the picture. No more of: 'It's me man, me alone against the world.' If this is your mind set, you better read my first book, and then come back to this one.

As we proceed along, there are many subjects that will come up, I will touch on them one by one, but for a full understanding, please seek additional literature on the subjects, for this is neither an encyclopedia or study guide, on Prevention. If anything, this book should be used more for a handbook or pocket book, a help book explaining the possibilities in the prevention field of addiction; and a reminder you are not safe if you use.

The Calling

Before we get into what I call the guts of the book, let me kind of present a starter, beginning, not sure if that is really what I should call it, but in lack of a better term I shall,—yet, if I had another choice I think I'd call it, "The Calling," because there is a hidden voice inside all of us alcoholics, and drug addicts;—this hidden voice gives this calling, most of us just drink more until it shuts up. But a few of us, and only a few I'm afraid, let it haunt us, until it wakes us up. And then, and only then, we can go to town and recover. This is what I call, "The Calling," oh yes, if you'll be quiet for a moment, listen, stop the drugs for a moment, the booze, it will call, you will hear it. Alcohol, it has its roots:

> *Arabic = 'al kobol' = "The finest of something."*
> *Latin = 'Spiritus Vini = "The Spirit of wine."*

In the Middle Ages—a great discovery was made, chemists discovered wine could be distilled, producing a very strong beverage known now as, Brandies, Whiskies, and Liqueurs. Before this great discover, man [and woman] had only wine and beer to contend with. Such a shame; in any case, from there came the deep human cravings we inherited [over simplified and under developed, but we get the jest of the matter, don't we?].

And then one day, an ancient Greek man wrote "Never walk at night and in the winter when you are drunk?" Why? I'm from Minnesota, and to me it is obvious, but let's goes back to the Greek. Let's look at his saying, his 'why'. It is said, he wrote these as his last words, meaning or indicating, he was to be buried somewhere on alien soil [while he was dying], and did not take a liking to that.

In winter time alcohol intoxication is very dangerous. And most people do not take preventive measures. I had a friend who was a boy-scout leader, mine to be exact. When I was about 20-years of age, I asked to somebody how he was still doing. His friend told me he had been out in the snow with a group of kids, being very heavy, he stopped to rest, told the other scout master to go on ahead, he'd catch up with them later, but he fell to sleep, and froze to death [I dare not say too much more on this matter, but everything has a price, and yes he liked his booze].

To be a drunk is liken to be a broken oar on Lake Superior in the middle of the night with a storm coming on. And so to you, my good friends, those who wish to sober up, throw away the crap, or is it crack, the storm is here, and you may be in that boat. The Ancient Egyptians knew that man or women were forsaken once they got a liking for the pleasures of drink, which did not remain sweet forever; yes, they knew plainly that hidden under the canopy of alcohol, is a curse, a curse that profligates, until total destruction appears.

Rosa's Story—From Peru

From my wife Rosa Siluk [and I shall quote her]:

"*Let me give you one more story, of my home in Lima, Peru, concerning a drunk. He was a lawyer, and when he used to drink, he never looked comparable to one, simply messy and out of sorts…out of reality, no dignity, acting and looking similar to a beggar. In any case, one night, and I capitalize on the word night, because it fits into the Greek saying my husband was talking about, and there in Lima it is not cold like in Minnesota, meaning, it was not cold, for in Lima it's warm and nice weather. Anyhow, one night this fellow was walking through the park, and he fell down, and was found dead the next day [and if there was to be anyone to help him, it most likely would have been during the day, not night] so like the Greek implied, night again seems to be in more dangerous when intoxicated.*

This thing called drinking is not only a North American subject, or Egyptian subject, or for that matter, a South American or Greek subject, it is a world issue, an international-global and ancient issue. And as my husband would say, you can be part of the recovery element, or part of the drinking issue. But like him, he now has been sober for 19-years, you can be part of the recovery element, and I am very proud he has buried it. I will never fully understand this problem because I'm not a user, nor ever was; but I believe what he says, because I've seen it in my country.

≈

I only want to share this second story with you because I do not want people to die, reminiscent of my brother [Augusto], who died because of alcohol; again it takes place in Peru. He started drinking when he was very young because issues he had, that he never seemed to solve. When he was 21 he stopped using alcohol, but it didn't do any good, he got cirrhosis of the liver and died. Now he would be 56-years old, had he made a different choice earlier on in life. But I know it is hard for young people to see this, it was for him.

    Thanks for listening to me, and I shall now return the book back to my husband.

    Note by the husband: *My wife was a little fearful about saying her brother was 21-and died of such a disease, and asked if she should mention it. I didn't give advice, rather facts and experience, saying, "Reality hurts, young people die also, maybe not as quick as older ones, but in some cases they do, and so no one can drink large amounts safely; no one, no one, and I mean no one.*

2

Similarities

✦

Sex Addiction vs. Alcoholism [part I]

This might seem to some, as they read on, that we are getting off the beaten path by presenting similarities between sex addiction people and alcoholic people, but if so only for a moment, or chapter. And I feel we need to look at some of the components we're talking about, if not for the afflicted, for the recipient of the behavior by the afflicted, or to make it plainer, the co-dependent.

On one hand it shows many of us may be in the same boat, called Addiction, and trying to jump over to the other boat, called Prevention and Sobriety, this might be good in itself. Having said that, let's look at the similarities between the two; we will first mention sex and the second comment will be referring to the alcoholic [in doing this chapter also, we can look at what behavior needs to be modified to bring the person out of his/her crisis, which in most cases is the reverse of what I am saying; also we may want to remember, prevention comes into play by modifying and not duplicating]

Sex Addiction vs. Alcoholism:

a.   Both try to alter one's mood [escaping and/or avoiding]; it is for both parties an analgesic [meaning, euphoria effect is sought].

b.   Both violate one's values

c.   Organism, equals =Substance intoxication [believe it or not]

d.   Both will sacrifice job, family, relationship loses

e.   Both have preoccupation components

f.   Both have urges

g.   Both have a loss of control

h.   Both have fantasies

i.   Both have disregard for consequences

j.   Both have imprinted images

k.   Both have affairs [one with the bottle, the other with flesh]

l.   Exposure=DWI' s [legal issues can be for both]

m.   Pornography [can be for both]

n.   Both have the experience [one the bottle, one the person]

o.   Both show unmanageability

Yes, we are resembling ducks in the same pond, we only look different outside and our actions may be altered a little, but inside we are both paddling up a water fall;—both hitting our heads against the wall. Both listening but not hearing, you know, going in one ear and out the other.

Belief System

Now let's look at the belief system, some of it will look like imprinted thinking [the blind following the blind one might say] and unmanageability. In many cases both parties [the Sex addicted and Alcoholic] believe in the same system, and in many cases the sex addicted is an alcoholic; let's see if you can point to something familiar, that is, let's see/review what excuses we used for our bad behavior:

1)   I'm not worthwhile

2)   No one cares about it

3)   It's a way to relax

4)   Sex is most important

5)   Sex makes isolation bearable

6)   It is needed for stress

7)   Just my needs

8)   Everyone likes it

The cycle is: 1) Preoccupation 2) Rationalization 3) Compulsion [act] and 4) Despair

Recovery: 1) Reverse alienation [establish a caring environment] 2) Find a new belief system and thinking 3) Work the 12-step program [to emerge from being a double pretender].

Levels [understanding what level you're in]:

Sex Addition:

Level One	=	Masturbation
		Homosexuality
		Prostitution Regarded as normal
		Heterosexuality
		Relationships
Level Two	=	Exhibitionism
		Voyeurism
		Indecent phone calls/liberties [illegal / victimized]
Level Three	=	Incest
		Child Molestation
		[Severe]
		Rape

Note: Life can be destroyed at any level

3

Similarities

◆

Gambling vs. Alcoholic behavior [part II]

Gambling addiction in many ways is similar to Alcoholism, both having alike criteria; for example, preoccupation, increased tolerance [meaning, tomorrow it will take more to give you the same mood altering affect your actions have today]. Also, both addictions have alike repeated efforts to reduce or stop. We see here a big control issue, despite the problems it is creating such as family, social and occupational issues.

I have worked with gamblers as well as drug addicts and alcoholics, the bad thing about the gambler, he can acquire his addiction a lot quicker than the alcoholic, believe this or not:—it is more psychological. Let's say 18-months for the gambler vs. 5-years for the alcoholic. You can put any kind of figures you want in place of mine, but the gambler and alcoholic know it takes a brief time to get psychologically hooked into the chase of gambling. For the counselor who says this is bullshit, go business and get some hands on research.

The gambler, similar to the alcoholic and addict share some essential features, such as: progression, no stopping power, preoccupation and disregard for the consequences. I think we heard that for the sex addict also, but again many of us are in the same damn boat. In point of fact, a compulsion to use/gamble at any cost is the premise.

In comparison to alcoholism, the gambler is more psychologically addicted I believe, or can be, I know I'm repeating myself, so what, listen, the destruction to relationships, social behavior and professionalism seem to be at the same level of significance with both addictions, as far as destruction goes. Oh, it's a hell of a merry-go-round. Stick with me, and we shall go around some more.

The Secret

There is something you may not know in this paragraph. So, please, read this very slowly. No, no, do not turn the page…not yet, for a great many Chemically Dependent folk, who get on to the recovery road, transfer their addiction to gambling. Oh yes, "WHY?" Is that what you are asking? I did a long time ago, that is to say, ask that very question. It is called the treatment centers do not teach what they should be teaching, because they don't know I suppose—know what? No problem, you will know in a second, without having to pay that treatment center $125 for an assessment. You get it for the price of this book.

Oh yes, when I worked for a freestanding facility many years ago, for every hour I talked to a person one-on-one, I made a check mark on a paper, and that paper with my name was given to the finance people, and the client was charged $100 for every check. Unbelievable, it must really be high now, not sure, I write books now, maybe I should go back to those check marks I made more money. Anyway, as I was about to say, many clients leave treatment sober but burdened with unresolved issues, with no solving techniques, character defectors and/or dual-disorders not checked [be it depression, anxiety or alike]. This person then steps into a world not knowing how to deal with his/her feelings [i.e. repressed anger/hurt, etc]. He avoids conflict, intimacy, hurt, and pacifies one's self with an escape [call it gambling]; this is called <u>disassociation</u>. If you are gambling in many cases this is exactly what you are doing;—avoiding issues:—trying to hide, when there is no tree to hide behind. It is like sitting in a meeting day-dreaming. That is what you are doing. Get off the pot, and stop it. You gave up one addiction for another that is all you did.

For those who are thinking about experimenting with this, let me bring a little more information to light. Please listen, you can read a little faster if you want, but don't speed read yet. When the new victim-to-be learns winning is a high, he also learns that he has to chase the loss [the no fun part], but continues none the less. Despair and panic is just around his/her corner. Anti-social behavior comes along for the ride, in the quest for a high; and it most likely is now an addiction. In many cases the alcoholic will relapse acquiring what we counselors call a cross-addiction [simply two addictions], to your learned experiences.

≈

We must remember, this book is about Prevention, and therefore, each chapter should be viewed with that being a pathway…in the above cases we have looked at similarities of sex, gambling and alcoholism, and many of its characteristics; but the end result must be to remain sober, or addiction free. And so remember what provokes might be a way for you to make a list of behavior you need to work on, a prevention list, plan. What to avoid. Call it a: *"Relapse Prevention Plan."* Under one line write "Undesirable behavior," if you wish;—maybe under another line you may want to put, "Times I'm most vulnerable", and make sure you are at the movies, or with friends during these weak times. For me I was always vulnerable between 7:00 PM and 10:00 PM, and so I've seen every movie in town. I had certain friends to call up—I asked them if I could call them when I was feeling the urge. I had a list of about seven people I could call. I had a list of AA and NA meetings of the whole city. Man oh man, this is no game, this is it? Life or death [I'm really trying to find some humor to put into this book but I'm failing in that area, sorry]. You can play around with this and expect to get away with anything, but it catches up with you, and will bite you right in the ass.

4

Behavioral Stages of Alcoholism

There are several stages to Alcoholism, and at this juncture, let's look and see where you may belong:

1. Pre Alcoholism Period: This is usually part of a gradual increase in drinking; finding more occasions to drink, experiences of feelings of freedom, adequacy and confidence [because of usage, you should have that without usage]; and it often turns into relief drinking for these people in this category.

2. Problem Drinking Period: This is a period one goes through where they find themselves constantly needing relief drinking [prior to alcoholism itself]; the person consumes greater amounts of alcohol than he did previously, and finds him/herself drinking by themselves [solitary drinking].

3. Pre Alcoholic Stage: This is a stage one really needs to counter; I consider it more of a transitional stage in the sense that you are at a point of no return when you find yourself gulping down drinks. But let me show the progression. First the drinker starts to get black outs, and may not even know it. Some people have had them for days, finding themselves in Paris or some far off land; believe it or not, when they wake up, have no recollection of the travel. Then the user graduates to hiding drinking, and to drinking before parties and social events, gatherings if you will;—now we are at the gulping stage, and you forgo social events, or use those events, to justify drinking, and if there is no drinking you avoid them. And on to Avoiding stage within this state, that is, talking about drinking comes about and again solitary drinking may get worse.

4. Acute Stage: This stage has to do a lot with physical and mental complications one gets from chemical usage. As one acquires these complications, they

contumeliously get worse;—such as having unreasonable behavior; confusion and frustration; always seeming to end up drunk; an overwhelming sense of guilt prevails, and extravagant behavior and the loss of esteem stagnate the person.

5. Chronic Stage: there is what is considered the early and late chronic stages in alcoholism; that bare many complications also. I have had a few friends of mine die because of this stage, and one in Vietnam: gastritis [farting oneself to death]; encephalitis [inflammation of the brain], also considered a water brain, you're fried my friend; nephritis [kidney] they can shut down eventually; and complications with the heart.

    > Note: I had recently learned of one of my old friends, whom I went to high school with, who got involved with drugs off and on, never ever able to quite kick the habit, went to prison, there he died of an overdose. It is very sad in that I remember him overly healthy. We fought, laughed and drank together. Actually several of my friends have ended up that way. Every time I go back to my old neighborhood I learn of a few more that have died from drugs or alcohol; all before their time.

    > *Note: for myself, I have had many of these physical combinations at times of my usage, and thereafter; and still have heart issues, had to have a bypass some 10-years ago;—had extreme problems for many years with gastritis. Had two strokes, and ended up with MS. I'm sure all in one way or another because of my 22-years chemical usage. We don't get away with much in life. So to the youth, time goes by fast, and you will find yourself with complications, like it or not, so stop while you're ahead, like my wife said in the beginning of this book.*

6. Early Chronic Stage: this is often marked by a change in attitude, no more concern about drinking, or responsibilities or for that matter one's activities. He/she shows disregard for family issues, and carries a lot of self-pity; often times he/she is hospitalized off and on; carries extra ordinary fears wherever he/she goes, and a decrease in sexual energy normally appears.

    > *Note [on my Mother]: Somehow I kept my job, paid my bills; that is until the very end, I call it round two. I sobered up for one year, then my wife still divorced me, and I went back to drinking, and lost my job, car and you name it, I didn't have it. Thank god my mother took me in, and let me*

sleep in her backroom of her apartment; otherwise I'd be dead today. I would have never made it back then, back in the 1980's. My mother has recently passed away, but she never made fun of my illness, or for that matter, took advantage of me because of it. She was a real mother, one with courage. And because of her, I am finishing this book; I was not going to, since I have one out on the fundamentals of Addiction, this being the follow-up one might say. But she pulled me through the hard times back then, and possible, this may help someone. I may never know. This book is the room, the back room my mother gave to me, take it my friend, while you can. People don't often knock twice at the same door. Thanks mom!

7.   Late Chronic Stage: in this stage if you got a friend I hope he kidnaps you, takes you to a hut in the middle of the Arctic, and sobers you up, if not you're a dead person waiting to be buried. In this stage the drinker is in total social isolation; is having prolonged benders; has a loss of morals, [that is to say, nothing will embarrass him at this stage]. He has increased tolerance [he either has to increase his drinking to get the same results, or if it is reversed-tolerance, he will use less for the moment because his system is saturated]; and last but not least he has what is called 'unnamed fears'. He is the living dead.

5

Discussion on Behavior: Trust

In the world of Prevention, "Trust is a Must,' why? If you want to skip to the last chapter and look at Prevention, it might help, otherwise let's simply look at the beast called trust first, and see where it might fit into Prevention, ok, for the why, will emerge; plus it is part of the secret I mentioned in the beginning of the book, you know, I said Prevention had its own little secret for success, well again, this is part of it.

I. Trust is—

Concept: trust is having a basic belief in the goodness of others [in addition to having a reputation of being a trust worthy person].

a)   Now let's put a little higher tone to it. It is also, a "Generalized Expectancy"

b)   Also, it is a "promise"

Both of the above ['a' and 'b'] are related to a group or individual.

Now let me make a few statements I believe in, and have found for the most part to be true: people who are high in trust are better adjusted psychologi-cally;—in general, everyone likes a trustier. Also, the more trust worthy a person is, the more moralistic the person is [and I say, usually], and is fre-quently involved in good works. And so being a trustful person, makes for a happier person, plus, prevention becomes more adaptable for the person, because the person is seeking a better life style;—the end result, the person, or persons have an improved chance in remaining sober.

c)   Being Gullible [easy to fool]. This is a touchy area while in the arena of 'trust,' but let's dig into it;—gullible in the trust world is not a nice word, it means believing or trusting in someone or another person's statement when there is clear cut evidence that the person cannot be believed.

My friend, this is not what trust is all about. You must tell this person you are not trust worthy, and if I were to trust you, I'd be simply gullible. In short, that is called prevention [and this is what is needed to be said]; from being gullible one might be lead into a relapse.

II. Trust can be Taught

Yes, you can teach yourself to be more trusting, simply follow the dots…

a)   Believe what your mate tells you; honesty in communication [belief, is trusting, unless you would be gullible, meaning, there is a good reason not to trust].

b)   You must gain confidence;—usually this is done by doing something over and over in a consistent manner; if you want to build trust that is.

c)   The parties that are working on trust must be together [how do you expect to work on something and not be semi-connected]

d)   Give consistent messages to each other [if you say you're going to the store, do not stop at the gas station, or pick up a paper, or stop and talk to George, Sam, Brenda or Diane—go home after your shopping is over; nothing like 'I told you so']

e)   If you do not trust, act as if you do and see what happens [or see if you can prove the person wrong, or prove yourself wrong] hopefully by trusting when you do not want to, your disbelief will be shattered by evidence that the person was trust worthy.

f)   There can be danger in distrusting, terrible things can happen. Often times the less trusting we become, the less trustworthy our own behavior becomes. Again this can be harmful to our recovery, and prevention outlook.

g)   We can model and encourage trust.

Conclusion to chapter five: High and low thrusters are capable of both being fooled; it might be wiser to trust simply because we are happier that way. And being happy is what recovery is all about, and it is what this book is all about, preventing us from going back to using, and trusting is simply one pain in the ass out of the way, so we can go forward.

6

Discussion on Behavior: Criticism

Often times during the process of healing, and working our program to remain sober, prevention comes in many forms. One thing, addictive people are real good at is, "Control". Yes, we normally end up having some horrific issues in this area. We want to control everything and everybody, but we are out of control,—are we not? Well, in a nutshell, criticism is a form of control believe it or not. And in the world of prevention, and Chemical Dependency, which you have chosen to venture into by picking up this book and reading it, Criticism, otherwise known as denigration [of the term I hate, which is belittling, but like to use] can get in the way of wholesomeness, that is, acquiring it, so what I am trying to say is work on it, I mean really work on it. But let's look at this beast a little closer:

1. **Control:** It is the art of verbal abuse and disapproval. Now for those wives out there who are trying to figure out why their husbands, boyfriends, sons or whomever, is always saying something to make you feel guilty, in a loud voice, swearing, and cutting you down all in one breath, this is called criticism, and he is using it to try and CONTROL YOU!!!!!!!!!!!!!!!!!!!!!!!!!!! Get it. Show him this paragraph................ Now if that person doing the cutting is looking at this it is you trying to control, YYYYYYYes YOU,—get off your high horse and get repaired, for you are damaged, and in need of help. Now to the other person, the one getting the scorn, you do not need to stand by and listen to his/her bullshit. If I were you I'd send the other person roses as a farewell gift, quick. If you allow the abuse-and control to continue, under the addiction umbrella, you will be sicker than the other person. What person with a healthy mind would stand by and allow the other person to scorn them forever and just bob up and done like a fishing line?

2. **Criticism:** Did you know, Ms. or Mrs. or Mr., this is a cause for depression-episodes? If you are a recipient of this criticism, get out of it; go to a hotel, or whatever you can do, do it; after awhile, when the damaged person is

working a prevention program [and has dealt with the control issue], you can consider moving back in slowly...yyyyyyyy, if that is what you want, after you find there are nice human beings out there, you may never want to go back. In any event, you only get more depressed at his expense while you stay under those conditions, and then come weaknesses, and heart attacks, and strokes, all that crap. No one is worth that bull.... Let dead dogs lay, for that is what they are when they do not seek help; yes, they are worthless to themselves, and any and everyone around them.

3.   **Power:** It is not the person who has the power to disturb you, nor is it the comment he/she makes. What does that above statement mean? Now your afflicted mate will want to see this, but do not show him or her yet. This is one of those areas considered "For your Eyes Only," [for either the dependent or co-dependent]:

You need to look at yourself—

a.   Overcoming fear of criticism [how!]

b.   Identify your negative thoughts [when being criticized]

c.   Analyze your thoughts for illogic or wrongness [remain calm]

d.   Comments right or wrong [if the comment is wrong forget it, if it is right you're not perfect, make the correction]

e.   Ask the question: "Do I need their approval?"

f.   Remember only your thoughts can upset you, therefore, think realistically.

> *Note: How you measure your thoughts is how you will absorb the comment. If you accept it as less than nothing, it is a worthless comment, a rhetorical statement. Pay no attention and go on your way; it is not worth your time. The more time you give it, the more worth you give the comment. Plus, on the Prevention Scale, you will notice it will not have the ability to provoke a relapse if you down grade the criticism to Zero; then get rid of the goofball.*

7

Discussion on Behavior: Triggers of Relapse

Anything that has the potential for triggering a relapse is a point of contention for *Prevention*. By and large, you need to work on it, eliminate it, and get rid of the unhealthy behavior [this is recovery my friend, no time to play games]:

1) Listen, look, and analyze what people are saying about you, doing around you. Why, simple, if you are too rigid, you may need to become a little more flexible.

2) If people are saying you react too quickly, emotionally, angrily, you may have to find out if there is a chemical in-balance in you; or if it is just the early stages of recovery, and you are relearning new emotions; that is, being flooded with several emotions at once and becoming overwhelmed by them. Check it out.

3) If you are not solving the problems you feel you should be in your recover process, you may need to practice focusing on issues and on one thing at a time.

4) If you are a caretaker, and most women are, they are in-born with this asset, if you will;—it is a form of rescuing people. They do not need care taking, or rescuing, rather nurturing. But what I was leaning towards is for you to learn how to "Let go…ooooooooooo," now.

5) If you are a yes person, practice saying no.

6) If you do not know how to be quiet, it's a good time to start.

7) If you are always being taken advantage of, get rid of those people, and find new ones, associate with those who do not take advantage [oversimplified, but to the point]

8) If you are an asshole, and fond of making trouble for everyone, but you're trying to improve, stop blaming and pointing fingers, behave, and listen, most asshole [like you] know about their high and mighty make up,—they got a good mental picture of just who they are,—snobs are snobs, you and I both know that, they just want the power to continue to be snobs, but we as recovering people do not want to continue with it; so let them drawn in their snobbery, and you and I improve.

9) If you can not stand angry people or arguing, learn how to, because it is costing you a hell of a lot to be a peace maker at any price.

10) Last, but not least, so I heard said, learn responsibility: "Everyone wants their rights, without responsibility," our recent, but not present, Minnesota Governor said that once, Mr. Ventura. Why, because it is part of being a damn man. Everyone wants to know nowadays, what is a man. The first thing is "responsibility". Don't worry about what the woman feels a man is, she doesn't know. And if you don't, you just learned one thing about being a man, responsibility. And when the woman says: "I'm leaving your ass for the guy down the street," let the bitch go, you know why, she doesn't want a man, and that is why she's hunting. The first step is for you to become all you can, under the sun. A good woman will pick up on that. There are not a lot of good men to pick from, so you will end up being a good catch once you do the work you need on yourself.

8

Discussion on Behavior: Self-Esteem

In this chapter we will look at self-esteem, in the world of prevention we need to know we are equal to the person next to us, that there are no differences in equality, but there are differences in roles. Having said that, which I should have saved for the end comments I feel, but wanted it to be up front, let's go into it deeper.

If you don't mind, I'd like to make three parts out of this chapter, if not for your clarity, for mine. I have learned in life to make things simple for myself, I get along with everything much better that way.

Part I

<u>Pieces of Self Esteem</u>

A) "Self Esteem" is:

a)   Self-worth

b)   Ego needs

c)   Human pride

B) "Self-Esteem" is:

Self-esteem, in essence hangs on the threads of the human hunger for dignity or honor or respect or regard.

It might be noteworthy, that the lack of self-regard [that is self-esteem] is usually in the form of antisocial behavior.

C) "Anger"

Often times anger is based on fear, that is, the feeling of being threatened, insecure, lack of self-confidence, which all comes from WHAT? Yes, you got it—low self-esteem [we fear because of the lack of control, and we have hurt underneath anger]. But let's look at anger with self-esteem closer.

Other things that come from low-self esteem are:

1)   Lack of trust [we just looked at this, how everything interrelates]

2)   Trying to prove yourself [self-approved]

3)   Shame [feeling inadequate]

D) "Self-esteem:—High/Low"

1)   Low self-esteem says: I have fears of commitments, and that solitude is too embarrassing [something that needs to be worked on]

2)   Negative Pride says: I don't need anybody; also, no commitments, or optimism [again, another area that needs to be worked on]

3)   Positive Pride says: I'm self confident, inwardly secure and non-defensive [all elements of prevention for the most part]

Note: the above areas need to be reversed, solitude can be good. We are complete with or without someone else, if you think not, again you need to work on this area. And in the world of pride, we all need people, as soon as we discover this the better.

Part II

Pieces of Self-esteem
That hangs on for dear life

The following things come from low self-esteem:

Faith= lack of trust which translates into-insecurity
Egotism= trying to prove you're somebody
Shame= disgrace

This all deals with having a poor image, or in support of, making a person have a poor image of "Self".

Part III

Emotions

Mending ourselves, Preventive Maintenance

In Prevention, we are working on ourselves to become the best person we can, if you are not, I'm not sure why you're reading this book. Prevention says I need to stop "Something" before it happens. Preventing it from happening; again the last chapter explains it better; by and large, to become this person, that you have set out to become [kind of reinventing oneself] you want to become, takes work, understanding and working on emotions, all part of the trip, the road map if you will. Part of the "Mending Wall," for so many of us have build walls around ourselves, walling ourselves in, and others out, silly isn't it, but we do it.

There are certain prevalent emotions that inflect our personality and destroy our self-worth, which is the same thing as self-esteem; these developing negative emotions block a person from developing, let me bring them forward, for they are all criminals [one must remember feeling and thinking are two different things].

Feeling is an emotion, thinking is a thought; we do not, or should not react to our emotions, we have them all day, and when we do—have them all day—we go up and down with them, up and down we will go, similar to a roller coaster; but we should not react to those emotions, rather, we should react to our thinking, that is why, we should think before we act, or react, that is [it makes sense, right?]. Now let's touch on a few troubling emotions, but first let me add, emotions are neither right nor wrong, they simply, just are:

1) Inferiority: feeling [sometimes thinking] you have no value;—replace it with "I, as a human being, have value" simple.

2) Depression: stops our motivation in life, you need to replace it with: "Dreaming the dreams that motivate you in life's-service"

3) Anxiety: stops our need for silence and meditation, replace it with "Silent security/meditation" [allow time for church, spirituality]

4) Guilt: blocks our mental system from putting away 'perfectionism'; reality says, "I'll do the best I can"

5) Resentment: stops our acceptance of other's imperfection; replace it with "Accepting other's imperfection"

6) Fear: blocks love or giving [fear is a feeling of danger]; replace it with love/giving [love destroys fear]

Conclusion note: Know that you are equal to the person next to you; also there are no differences in equality, but there are differences in roles.

9

Resistance and Co-dependency

This chapter will be quite small compared to the previous, but in the few lines I will offer, remain a big importance, for with resistance, not much can get accomplished.

Resistance: is a fear, or put it another way, defense not to get close. In this case, resistance can involve denial, deletions, distortions and generalizations; I call those little white lies; in essence, one tells the self: you do not have to do what you must. You see, we played the game so long, and fooled so many people, we ended up playing it with and by ourselves, but now to ourselves we can fool without hinder, interruption: Why—no one else wants to play anymore. In prevention, we can not nurture resistance.

Resistance blocks the natural process to **Change** [Prevention]

Resistance is a defense not to get close, a fear

Resistance breeds resistance [that is, whomever you throw it upon, expect to get it back in your face]

Elements of Resistance: Control=insecurity [which is a feeling of being unsafe]; insecurity=fear [which is a lack of trust]. That is why we must work on all the elements in this book, one connects to the other.

Advise: Go with the flow, it is all you can do, if you are a counselor, or onlooker, break it by using immediacy= a challenge.

Co-dependency

Bottom line, co-dependency is "The loss of self". I really need not say anymore, but I will. There have been tons and tons of trees cut down to write about this subject called co-dependency. When in essence, it is not all that complicated; or at least that is how I see it. But let's look at this creature for what it is worth:

A) Co-dependency often belongs to your mate, in a relationship—but, can also belong to you, the addicted, or slave to the habit.

B) Co-dependency says: your partner is addicted to you, as you are to the substance [alcohol, gambling, sex, or drugs].

C) When all a person can talk about is his/her partner, consider that person Co-dependent.

D) **Relationships of the Tri-Circle:** Here is a kind of mental graph game. Try to visualize it, if you will. In circle one of these relationships you will only find one person fully in the circle [draw a circle on a piece of paper if you want, I can wait......ok, now], the other person, person two is half in and half out of the circle, not like person one who is in the circle fully [waiting for the other person to arrive, so we will see how he or she arrives], making that second person not quite in the full circle—whole [meaning he is only half a person in the circle], and therefore, co-dependent [on his mate; but the person fully in the circle is not co-dependent but rather, can be interdependent]. In circle two [draw another circle now], you find both persons in the circle [draw two people in the circle please] but interconnected, making them inner dependent; some say this is healthy, some say not healthy enough though. In the third circle [draw another, I know, you're getting tired, but if you're not visual, this is best] you find both of the people fully in the circle not touching one another or connected and this is considered healthy. This allows each person to fully grow at his or her speed, and able to distinguish bad from good, should one become unhealthy, the healthy one can get out. Thus, if you are joined too tight together like in circle two, or halfway in, like in circle one, your guess is as good as mine, we fall into the concept of allowing others to make our decisions for us, and of course, in many cases, they make decisions that are good for them, not necessarily for our benefit.

Conclusion: Seek your higher power [God]; let go and go forward in your life; and last but surely not least, and maybe I should have put this first, find a good 12-step program, and work the first three steps quickly.

10

Adult Children of Alcoholics [ACA's]

I do not care to elaborate too much in this area for we have briefly talked about co-dependency and in a like manner ACA's follow a similar pattern. Inasmuch as, co-dependency can occur in many ways and forms, ACA's may find their descriptions of behavior parallel. And we can go as far as to say, they are two peas in a pot. Prevention in this area might reside in the fact you need to own your own behavior, get out of denial, and modify undesirable behavior. Something that seems to be repeated over and over in this book, and so I will not repeat it so much here, but first...

first if you sense some of these characteristics belong to you, and you have an alcoholic parent, then you need to seek recovering for your freedom. In the long scheme of things, you can make your recovery process, and/or assets as soon as you claim your freedom. Some of the behaviors you may find here may or may not belong to you in the following areas:

1) Control issues;—not only with yourself but control of the feelings and behaviors of others. This is really called 'Fear of losing control,' one might add.

2) One might call this area of thought 'buried feelings,' that is to say, having a flat affect. Often times anger and sadness is withheld as a child, thus the ability to feel or express is thin at best. Again fear plays a roll in this dilemma.

3) Conflict. In this area we find fear, again it plays a huge role, but this time the person is usually fearful of people with authority; or angry people [anger can be used as a tool for the opposite party to get control of you]. In any case, as a result, the person avoids conflict, because of the fear factor. You see that is not approval, the very thing they seek. Make sure you do not find a place to hide, many do. Learn how to face what you have to. Become assertive

without becoming aggressive. There is a difference. Aggressive is attacking; being assertive is saying and doing what you need to do, no more, no less.

> ***On a personal note,*** *One of my ex-wives had a hard time dealing with anger. And so her ex-husband [not me] and her two children knew how to win every fight with her, just get angry at her and you won the fight. Again, it is a control tool. Maybe what you need to tell yourself is that, anger is a natural emotion, and people are allowed it, as you are. And if they want to express it, it's fine. If they want to displace it on you, it is called abuse, and it is not fine. Tell him/her, you are trying to control me by anger-persuasion tactic, and that is wrong; it is wrong because you are not being allowed to act in a free manner. If they disrespect that, they disrespect you; tell them to f-off [sorry about the F word, put for once it fits].*

4) Responsibility. Oh yes, we got to bring out the big one again. The big hammer that is, the thing nobody wants to hear or do. But you can't have rights without responsibility, our ex-Governor said it, and if he ever said anything, this to me was the one thing he was 100% right in. Normally ACA's and Co-dependents have this over-developed sense of responsibility;—especially women, who want to caretaker a person. I know women are born with these care taking-characteristics, but you must learn to nurture, not caretaker. The difference is, in care taking you walk for the person, in nurturing, you teach him how to walk. Don't put on his shoes my dear friends. And if you do put on his shoes and walk for him, I'd work on self-esteem.

A Last Note:

Life is never easy in recovering, working on prevention, trying to remain sober. Trying to deal with emotions, the thinking process, becoming the person you were meant to become. But you know, it is life, it is what it is all about. This is it, our stage, our world around us, or time. And so the four areas I mentioned above are but a few areas that are lying on the table for ACA's and Co-dependents to look at, and let me add a few more so you have something to look forward to, how about: feelings of guilt, inability to relax, harsh self-criticism, denial, relationships being quite difficult for you; a little food for thought. If these areas are issues for you, you need to work on them.

11

My Philosophy on Prevention

✦

[For Clients and Counselors]

Everyone thinks a little different, although in many cases, especially in the helping fields of humanities, akin to Chemical Dependency Counseling, we have similarities. And that is why I have called this last section "My Philosophy on Prevention," it may differ from others, yet I sense it is not all that different than my colleagues. Having said that let me provide below my statement to you; it may be a little complex, but bear with me; incidentally, the secret I mentioned is right around the corner, I think you already know it though.

Prevention can come through many channels, such as the school system, the community, the family, the one-on-one counselor. Early identification can give potential abusers an alternative or stop a potential crisis. My belief is that a Prevention Specialist, or counselor for that matter, should have some knowledge and/or experience in four models of prevention;—as to help his client. Not having these the client should, I believe, seek another counselor who does. The client can check the "helpers" resume out, that is to say, where he acquired his training, knowledge and/or experience, such as internships, schooling, etc. Ask him or her, or ask their bosses what is his background.

Now you may be asking, "What have I used in providing my clients information…?" In the Socio-cultural, I've used lectures to DWI recipients. In a like manner, I advise people seeking Prevention tools to seek out good lectures in maintaining sobriety. At hospitals I have worked at, I've used the social psychological approach using educational tools to include 'Distribution of Consumption,' model with both in-and-outpatient clients.

<u>**The Public Health Model**</u>;—as I have stated in a number of ways in this book and my previous book on sobriety, in the area of <u>**Prevention**</u>, my belief is, in a nutshell, is to use 'whatever means it takes to bring about sobriety [legal], to prevent a potential alcoholic or drug addict from using, or for that matter bring

an end to an addiction related crises; yes, I will do whatever it takes to do this, as you should. Remaining sober is a process, if need be we must, break the blocks of denial, over and over, creating change in our drug of choice. Prevention requires effort, and this effort reduces the outcome of alcohol and drug use in a monumental way.

For me the Health Model is simply, to help the person become all he/she can. Meaning, as a counselor my job is to help you become, and as a client your responsibility is to become, as healthy as possible, in a round-about way [this circle of recovery involves, social, psychological, spiritual and physical health]. Again I stress, your goal and mine should be for you to become as wholesome as possible.

Client & Counselor

This is why it is so important for the client to pick out a good qualified counselor, he is helping you reshape you, and he the client is counting on it to happen. He/she [the counselor] should be directing you to a variety of areas [this book could be one]. But let me go beyond this book: predominantly I've used the 12-steps in the past, and preach them; give or have AA lists, Aftercare and continuum of care outlets should be available for the client, co-dependency groups can be recommended for the client, confidentiality in the area of one-on-one counseling must be kept, and insure you as well as your clients have friends to talk to.

Learn the disease concept to understand your make up. Learn early identification of your traits. Learn the difference between in and out patient treatments, to see what you may need if you predict a relapse. If you are not sure where you are at in the addiction stage, or what the word means, seek a pre-assessment: finding out if you are an abuser or dependent. Get a healthy attitude. Learn coping skills, cues, or signs for yourself. Education can mean salvation my friend.

Treatment and prevention often look alike, and in some ways are inseparable, I believe. Usually treatment has a consequence, prevention does not. Prevention is preventing the occurrence of usage, chemical usage, as treatment is in itself, treating the user in a controlled program.

Prevention programs can help identify problems before they become severe, or should be able to;—again it is the program and the counselor, the client needs to look at, plus the client can not be resistant, let go and go forward, do not forget that phrase, quote it everyday if you have to: "Let go, and go forward"—that is the end product. There are three areas of prevention, hang on to your seats and thinking hats, we are going into a new zone, but you need to know what they know—the counselors, a little bit anyhow. There are good, very good counselors out there in this field, do not be afraid, or intimidated to seek one out. They are not gods but they do their work, in most cases, and have his blessing. You have to work in this field.

12

Prevention Zones

Zone One: Primary Prevention. You need to operate on a level that will alter the set of opportunities; risks and expectations surrounding your environment as a whole [use it before abuse occurs]. Example, get government and/or public education regarding your addiction [learn all you can]; you've got to be changing your customs, values, and norms; presenting alternatives for drinking, or taking drugs,—for personal growth.

Remember the old saying, "No pain no gain," simple dedication, and the lazy man is out. It is like everything in life, how bad do you want it? That is the big, big, big, big, big question. Mother Teresa once said about a potential new student who wanted to be trained by her, with her, but Mother Teresa after receiving her letter of introduction and request, never responded back to the student's letter. A reporter, who knew this, asked Mother Teresa why she never did, and she said something to the effect: If the student really wanted to be here, she would be here. In a like manner, in 1968, I was studying Karate in St. Paul, Minnesota. Everyone talked about the Master Karate man Gogan [The Cat] Yamaguchi, and his son Gosei. And so I travel 2000-miles to learn from him, and we became very close friends during this period of my life in San Francisco. And all the ones who thought about it back in Minnesota in my dojo [gym] were of course left out. And so, if you want it bad enough, you will get it. No game playing with yourself. Don't waste everyone's time if you really do not want it.

Zone Two: Secondary Prevention. This area of prevention, it is supposed to identify people in the early stages of chemical dependency. It is more focused on a select group [respectfully];—for the client and counselor, we're looking at early identification for individuals who have potentially harmful family drinking histories. If you have, you may have to pull away from them to maintain sobriety. And as a counselor, you may have to tell them so,—but you must believe in it, for it is his/her life. I would not hesitate to tell the person to keep his or her distance from a family that abuses or uses alcohol, if need be. Matter of fact, I would confront them directly and let them know where you stand, or I stand, and although you may love them, going back to usage is not an option, they must go before you start using; you can simply tell them, "I can not be around you…" point blank. No jokes, this is serious business. Like it or not. Don't worry, they really do not want to be around you most likely if you are not using anyhow. To them you will simply be a dead-beat watching them get drunk, and no one wants a guard standing by.

If you can't say that, then go get drunk, high, there is much more pain out there waiting for you. And have a happy and miserable death with your loved ones for you're all going to die before your time. Matter of fact, throw this book away, it is not going to do you a bit of good with that attitude. Nobody, I mean nobody out there cares Mr., about you getting fucked up as much as you, so don't expect the bar tender to have sympathy, he doesn't, it is not what he is getting paid for. Watch your friends fade into the long lost sea, as you sober up.

Zone Three: Tertiary Prevention. It is a fancy name for a counselor to use, so the client can't understand it I think. You know one of those things when you ask about prevention, and he says, "Oh yes, we will have to use Tertiary Prevention on you," then he gives you a $100 an hour bill. Not sure what this book cost yet, but you get the same information for the price of the book, and it is not $100-dollars. Good deal right?

Tertiary Prevention is a basic grouping, trying to end compulsive use of alcohol [in other words, addiction per se]. Let's look at it a little closer. This area of prevention measures, or could measure I should say, the contaminate level of a person's intoxication. Let me try and explain it in a different light. It tells or should tell a person he or she needs detoxification or institutionalization. It is used for a chronic person who is modeling or showing bad social influences. An example might be, or was when Billy Carter, Ex President Jimmy Carter's brother went out to get on a jet, and stopped by one of the wheels [landing gear] to take a piss; this was live on TV, and the whole world seen it. This was a chronic alcoholic who was modeling contaminated social influences. Sorry that's the best I can do with that big word "Tertiary."

Conclusion

In the world of addiction, such as: alcoholism and drug abuse, along with the many other addictive psychoactive drugs, like caffeine, smoking, etc. and eating disorders, gambling, sex, etc. One must remember who he or she is listening to; and for the counselor, who he or she is talking to. By and large, women's groups are different than child's groups and one might have more genetic components involved, also ethnic factors play a part in prevention. And to take this to other level, age groups, such as, the 20's think different than the 40's groups. In this world of prevention, it is not the old or new, not what is good for the goose is good for the gander, quite the opposite, the truth is, we are all different, and all need truth, and a way out of this mess of addiction. What is good for the gander might be foolish for the goose. Remembering we are different, and may need different cures, can be helpful, as in some cases of homosexuality, bi-sexuality, etc.

Once a black-woman, about 30 said to me, prior to a one on one session, our first session to boot, after finding out I was her counselor, she said: "Now what can a white, older man do for me, you got to be kidding." She had a good point, and I needed to answer her question. You see, all counselors need to answer questions. You can tell the difference between a good counselor and a great one. The good one will be learned, like the great one, the great one will have it "in born" he is born with the skill, and he will always have the answer; maybe not the one you want, but it will be 9 out of 10 time, the right one. And when it is not right he will walk away, let you know, and most likely say, "Educate me". How do I know, well, because I'm one of those great counselors, believe it or not. I have always had the answers, almost automatically.

If I was talking to a Prevention women's group, I might be talking to them about the high risk factors such as cancer, suicide rates, and death from scleroses, in comparison to men. One thing all groups need is to be taught discrimination.

Moreover, prevention I believe should attack a conglomerate network to include your health, illness, and the causes that may lead to death; behavior effects such as paranoia, apathy, depression, intellectual impairment, and nutrition. In addition, proliferation of adolescent crisis to where their social skills are hindered should not be excluded. So parents look; and counselors, include.

In closing, you being the client, or the wife, or husband of the inflicted, your counselor should be an advisor, advocate, consultant, teacher, in addition to a counselor. And his job, as well as the individual's job is to harness a potentially wild horse before it looses control and gets outside the corral. I would say good luck, but let me change that to say, God Bless.

◊

The Secret

People are not the same, and it is silly to think one race or culture can use prevention the same way another can. I grant you, you must leave no stone unturned when you are in your pursuit of achieving the ultimate in sobriety, in the training of your body. With this issue, nothing can be overlooked. Likewise, you can neither live for, or in the past, but keep seeing new methods in keeping yourself from old habits. All this is Prevention in a nutshell. Although everything is important in Prevention, and some things more so than others depending again on the race, culture, gender, age, etc. One thing, "The Secret", is the most important, when all is said and done: that being, again it is not practical to think everyone must do it the same way. Your Prevention Plan should be adaptable to you, not to anyone else. As I have also mentioned in this book and my previous one on addiction, "What ever it takes, do it."

Prevention is a fight to the end, in saying that let me share an experience: I had taken up karate in San Francisco [1969], in the late 60's with the famous Gosei Yamaguchi, and his father, whom I met, was none other than the distinguished "Cat", Gogen Yamaguchi. And I had learned back then in studying karate a secret, and now as a counselor, I have relearned the same secret, after all these years, and in all my studies at the four universities I attended I have learned a secret, one thing among everything else stood out for success—*balance*;—in college it can be simply sitting in the right seat so the professor can see you, it helped back then, believe me; sometimes it is more simple than you think; yes a balancing act of getting to know him or her, could be it. The teachers often would look for you, and some people would be sitting elsewhere, but I'd be right there. It helped me in more ways than one can imagine, if anything, to get to know the teacher. And of course, sleeping well, and eating right helps the thinking, the mind becomes balanced. In karate, we learned many things, the Cat Stance being one [or a battle stance], but all in all, we learned how to rest the body in a perfect balance; thus, the movements to follow, went with the laws of physics, and gave me the time to apply more speed in relationship to my mind and body's needs, call this balance my friend. And in the Army, of which I spent eleven years, again I witnessed "Balance," in play, conformity, unity, balance in cadence in marching, in marksmanship, in everything. I was a Staff Sergeant when I got out. In any event, balance came in handy then, and it still does, even as I am writing this book, it has to have balance. Let me also add to this writing on balance, it was especially needed in Vietnam where you needed to balance emotions with thinking, and do it quick:—and trust your senses, a balancing act to say the least.

In a like manner, Prevention is stopping something before it happens. And when it comes down to the wire, you must use all the skill and wisdom available to you. There are no tricks here. You can not go into this blind, and expect to come out with the whole picture; that is to say, you can not be a blind man touching a horse's ass,—for in describing it as to being a horse although your intent would be right, your picture would be wrong. And again, the picture in Prevention can not be wrong. If truth is missing in your heart to go on this adventure into Prevention Land, stay home and get drunk, you will not make it; go play with the blind man. Only in that totality can you find this balance, its true picture to be.

—The secret in Prevention is "Balance".

13

Overview of the 12-steps

I can't remember how many times I went into AA or some support group and they were talking about the 12-steps. Sometimes they were working on step one, or step five, or step ten. They all seemed to know what they were talking about, but when I asked them, afterwards in the coffee room, they could only related to step one, four or ten. Why I asked myself. Could it be they didn't learn them properly? Grabbed the first three and said hell with the rest. Let me explain in a quick review how I see them. For in recovery it helps to understand everything underneath, hiding, that is, under the surface.

Step one; is considered one of the God steps; read it at your leisure, and as you do, you will see its character is imbedded in power, yes, yes, yes, power, power, and more power. The first three steps deal with god, so we call them Control or God Steps. What are we really saying in these three steps? Here it is in a nutshell. If you do a good first step and a bad third step you might just as well start all over. Step one you admit, step two you find faith, and in step three you find hope. Within these three interlinking steps you find out your life is 'unmanageable,' and if you don't, you haven't worked them. Put the book away, and go get plastered, because you are about to, anyways. Then come back when you are ready to admit your life is 'unmanageable.'

We're still on the first three steps so don't go avoiding this paragraph, get back here. Now let's take the power, and god, and name these steps 'Higher Power Steps'. Why? Because your life is unmanageable, and you need someone bigger than you to put it back together, like Humpty-dumpy, one might say;—in a like manner, I guess you could say, when you do say, 'my life is unmanageable,' you are—at that point—acknowledging, say again, acknowledging insane behavior on your part.

Now who is your higher power? Since you may not believe in God, pick out a noun=person, palace or thing. That will do for the time being.

So you see the first three steps is like the *'Three Musketeers,'* all for one and one for all, sort of anyhow.

Now let's call them the <u>Decision</u> steps;—for are you not at a point of trying to make a decision? Yes you are, and by the time you finish these steps, you should have made your first big decision; if not, you need more pain. I know I keep saying this, but it just is not going to work without the 'willing'; stop fighting this, you got to let go and go forward; the fighting is over, over, over, over…got it, it is OOO—VER!!.

Step Four: Here we go again. Someone says: "Let's work on step four" and you get confused with steps 5, 6, 7, 8, and 9,—why? There is really a good logical reason for this, because they are all interconnecting steps [making them look similar]; oh yes, don't get mad and throw the book down and say these other people are teaching me wrong [in my book "Aftercare," the 12-steps is explained in more detail, if these paragraphs are not enough information for you]. They are teaching you the way they know, as I am. When I used to do group therapy, I would always give this sermon first, and then the next day starts with the steps. And if a person came in late, I'd give them a hand out explaining this, and have him explain it to me later on, and sometimes in front of the group, and if he couldn't I'd have to give another lecture in this area somewhere along the line because I'd know the person who came in late would not get the idea of the whole three parts of the steps [being, the control steps 1 thru 3, the action steps, 4 through 9; and the maintenance steps 10 thru 12]. Having said that, let's remember the three first steps where you made your first decision in this program, connect with the bottom lower six action steps, where you put the decision into practice, and both the action and control steps have to be maintained, or polished, and so we got the last three steps that connect with the two upper sections, in doing just that. You see, it's becoming easier, I hope.

Now let's try and connect these six action steps together. These are all called action steps. Let me repeat: action, action, action, action, action. I always do that when I want to memorize something. I say it five times.

Step four [#4]; you got to make an inventory. Step five; you got to admit to god, and a friend or someone of your wrongs, get it out. Find someone understanding, not judgmental. Step six; you should now kind of know your issues, problems, defects or behavior you want modified, change. These are the things you learned wrong, and consequently, need to relearn right, again. So this step called #6 is like 4 and 5, is working on the things you glued to your personality, character if you will, long ago. For example, envy, anger—remove them, ask your higher power [from step one] to cut them out of your mind, flesh. Have you ever seen, or heard of people talking of a certain people who say he's stop drinking but…, "He stopped drinking but keeps on talking with that same old rotten mouth of his, and still has bad character" [?] Well my friend, he worked the first three steps, and got lazy and didn't work on the next six action steps. YES, he is sober, but he is acting like a 'Dry drunk,' which is a person who has stopped drinking, but has the same old behavior. He needs to work the 'Action Steps,' not only the three control steps. By not doing this, he will be a recovering alcoholic with the old alcoholic behavior, God help his family.

You need to realize your defects. Sometimes these hidden defects, or unwanted behaviors are called 'blind spots,' because you do not even know you have them, or that in the above case, you're talking silly [rotten that is, and unaware of this]. So at this juncture, three or four people are saying: "Hay, what the hell you are talking about," stop and think,—listen to what these people are really saying [they are saying you are a sober drunk], maybe you need to work on a certain area. Be true to yourself by being upfront with yourself;—if you do not want to fix yourself up, so be it, that is your business, and we, or for that matter, no one can make you, but don't pretend, pretence is a waste of time for everybody, it is just working against the grain, spitting in the wind one might liken it to, and you start to take it out on everyone around you. Say your goodbyes and be honest with everybody, you've given yourself enough grief throughout your using life,—along with everyone else, we've all [they all I should say] got a stomach full of you, and you got a stomach full of you, go and die in peace. And you do know that is the next step, #13. Nevertheless, these 'Action Steps' is a gateway to the last three steps called the "Maintenance Steps," or "Prevention Steps."

Step Ten: Actually we worked through these steps quickly, haven't we? See I told you so. You may say, why doesn't he put down the actual working for the steps? First, you need to do some work, if I put them down you'll have me doing the work, this is unfair and I will not be abused. Second, when you learn a language, you talk in that language. That my friend is what we are doing now, talking in the step language, and very few people know this language, usually only counselors. When someone says let's work on step two, what first comes to mind? Think about it before you read on.......................got it, it should be 'Higher Power Steps,' then you should say to yourself, 'these are all linked to Decisions." Now when you go to steps 4 through 9, what should you say? The man says, "We are working on step seven today." Think again...............got it? You should be saying something like, 'Action Steps, these are action steps, therefore, I got to work on behavior.' You may not be able to define the actual step, but you know what highway you're on. Before you were lost in the cloverleaf, got the picture? For example, let's say a person says at AA or NA, we're working on step '8', now you can't quote it but you know it's an action step [I repeat], and it is linked to step 5, and that step 8 and 9 are linked together pretty tight. In any case step 8 means you got to make a list of people you harmed and 9 indicates you should make amends.

Now you go back to 5, admit to a friend, remember we talked about that. Now let's look at step 4 which is linked to step 5, 6 and 7 which are linked pretty tight together. Step 7 indicates you got to remove your defects, but 6 indicated you came to a realization, and 1, 2, and 3 you made a decision to go forward on with this healing process, and that you couldn't do it alone. You see how the first three blend into the action steps? I know we're supposed to be on the last three, 10, 11, and 12, so let's blend in [I get carried away sometimes].

When you buy a house it doesn't stop there, you got to mend fences now, right? Sure you do. Just like in recovery. This is why we call this book 'prevention'. And steps 10, 11, and 12 are just that—preventive in nature, simple. In these steps you continue to take YOUR inventory, not your neighbor's, or mother's, or wife's or brother's—just, yours, yours alone, yours, yours, and only yours alone— we like taking other people's inventory, and pointing fingers, don't we? Oh sure we do, we use the "but's," and the "if's" real well [you know what I mean, "If only I had the chance," or you may hear, "But you don't understand."] We understand real good, once we sober up, and we know addicts and alcoholics are professional liars, they can manipulate so good, it is unbelievable, they've had enough practice they should be good. Matter of fact, we spend more time perfecting our treasured bad behavior, we got little time for comforting others. But we have to, it is life or death with us, right, we got to have that drink, or that fix. The square person doesn't understand this, and this is why you and I could fool them. They kept thinking we were predictable, and had limits in what we'd do, but we fool them, we went far beyond those limits. Maybe even selling, or hocking our wedding rings, does it hit home. How about taking money out of a loved one's purse, or pocket, haw; oh I know you know what I'm talking about. You may not be saying it but you're thinking, 'been there, done that,' but in a different way.

What is an inventory? It is what is happening with you, what is happening in your life. YOU are the inventory. Yes, for once it is all about you, you, just the way you like it. Are you still envious? Are you still walking downtown saying, "Mother Fucker, mother fucker," you know, that great vocabulary that you picked up in the bars, in the alleys, while telling your friends how tough you were, you got it now, right, the tough guy syndrome, we all get it, it's not your invention, should you be so damn arrogant and think it is—try and get back to being a human being, not a sponge. If you are not out of the 'Mother Fucker,"

stage, you are not working the last three steps. Now don't tell me how hard it is, I already know, just work it, you will find no pity down this lane, this is 'Pitiless Lane,' my friend, you got to walk it, but not necessarily alone. If you can go hunting, bowling, to movies, to work, screw at night, if you can put out all this energy, you can work the last three steps.

Step's 11 and 12, indicated you will need ongoing support, meditation prayer,—this will help keep up the spirit within you, plus guide you, in case you start shifting to bad thinking, also known as, 'stricken thicken'. And the last step, as a result of doing this workout of sorts, you need to help someone else, stretch out your hand, it will not fall off, don't be so tough. A king once said: he got better results from being humble and gracious than from being strict and unwavering. If you have made it this far, God bless you, you have worked a hell of a program, and you, yes, you are one of the few lucky ones that got this far. If you got this far and have not made a decision to work this program, to stop your usage, God bless you none the less, but stay away from me. I work with the willing, not the silly. Only 1.5 % of true addicts and alcoholics make it this far, this far meaning, to a sobriety status, which last over two years. You can be one of these people, right now, celebrate if you have, celebrate if you're going to start. If you can't you will celebrate anyway, but it will not be my way. If you have stopped, or are stopping, and you can't for some odd reason celebrate your non-usage, you got to work on that also, it is called shame [people with shame find it hard to celebrate, shame is feeling there is something wrong with you]; it's all part of a tune up my friend.

14

Drugs and Poisons

Let's take a quick look into the world of drugs and poisons. It might be rousing to know, poisons start with plants, and same as drugs do, just like your drug. And we can look at psychoactive drugs, such as tea, coffee, tobacco, for instance. And then we can shift to more hazarded drugs such as alcohol and narcotics. Let's point to hashish, opium, cocaine, morphine, and heroin; the most prevalent of today. But also let's look at venomous pets, such as scorpions, snakes, millipedes. In the world of prevention, do we not poison ourselves in the long run? Is that not how we die, killing ourselves little, by little, while our, our internal organs rot away. If you think not, you have fooled even yourselves.

This area of poisons is seldom mention in books, not sure why, it is one of the most preventive-needed reviews in the whole spectrum of substance abuse and/or dependence.

And so what do poisons do? They paralyze; such as hemlock [prussic acid]; found in Europe [I will come back to this a little later possible], but did you know Socrates drank hemlock [Ciruta Virosa] and died from it, a plant known as cowbone, the toxin in this plant is virulent and horrifying in its affect, the form he used was the spotted hemlock, not water hemlock, which is a convulsive poison. In any case the first systems in the poison cicutoxin, takes 20-minutes to bite you. The mouth and throat will burn, abdominal pain comes, nausea, a sense of intoxication takes over, dimming vision occurs, and drowsiness;—the suffer becomes helpless, and feeble—you do not escape its crushing forces. In either case, both are killers; and after these symptoms are used up, then come another symptom called convulsions. I use this as an extreme example that drugs can be used wisely to help, or unwisely to destroy a system, and most can be put into the category of poisons, especially if used wrong.

Curare—arrow poisons. We find poisons in red beans from Mexico; from potatoes, tropical thorn apples. Botulinus—bacteria bring instantaneous death; poisonous fish: such as, dogfish, sting rays, river eel, worms and snails, the common toad, bees and wasps, and Spanish fly.

All these poisons can be a blessing or a curse, and some can be weapons such as mustard gas used in WWI, "x" poisons, yperite, vomiting gas, chloropicrin, thilone—worse than the side effects of the atomic bomb; nerve gas, sarin, soman.

And so I bring these drugs only to your attention so we can look at the whole picture of chemical substances available, abused, and used, and which we die from.

Notes by the Author

For the most part, these notes are brief at best, possible too brief, but I felt I should put them in for clarity sake, and for those interested in a little more detail in this overwhelming-mirage called addiction and prevention:

Notes: 1-On Thinking and Confusion: The drunk says, "Why can't I remember?" This happens more frequently than you think, especially to those who have had a long history of alcoholism, or for that matter, not so long history with PCP. In any event, the drunk says, "What?" His trouble is in thinking, the brain, and I'm sure you already know this, and if you do, so let it be a reminder. But as I was about to say, repeated usage will fry your brain, or put a different way, water it down to where you can not think. It's not you getting old that is doing this 'memory loss,' thing, it is simply the effects of not allowing the brain to repair itself. And after a certain point of time, some people's makeup never can repair the loss.

Notes: 2-On Street Living: I once read a Medical Doctor, who wrote a book on alcoholism, say all the alcoholics are living on the streets. How untrue this is. I was an alcoholic; I never slept, or lived on the streets. Matter of fact, all the alcoholics I knew, never did. Grant you, there are many who do. But let's look at it for what it is worth. If you want to drink, you work, and you hide the fact you are an alcoholic. I did it for 17-years, and then I got to the chronic stage, yet I still did not live on the streets.

The truth of the matter is, a very small percentage live on the streets, and the rest are living right next to you, your neighbors, your friends, your world leaders, your singers, and writers, and artists, and your loved ones. They are in your churches and at your job location, working next to you.

Notes: 3-On Books on Prevention, Aftercare and Support, Addictions: I've been to several bookstores, and I'm quite surprised to see there really is not much on Aftercare, and Prevention, and just a little on Addictions. This has provoked me to write a third book on this subject, called "A Path Through Aftercare," be looking for it.

Notes: 4-On Recovery and Limitations: Some people believe quite the contrary to what I'm about to recommend, or suggest to you, but so be it, they need to live it, and most of the people I've read or heard it from have no-hands on experience. In any case, let me explain, the first couple of years of recovery, make life simple for yourself so you do not have to make big life choices, work on remaining sober instead. For the early recovering person, what we [the person who has many years of recovery, myself included] call normal, rational and healthy choices are not confusing, but can be for the early recovering person. During my first years of recovery I took a part time job, then a full time job, just to acquire more sanity, clarity in thinking, learning how to deal with emotions. This might not be possible for you, but none the less, try to avoid the bumps in the road, or facing trials not necessary. Solving problems of recovery are of utmost importance. Again, try and make life simple, you can gradually jump into the ocean later. Reminiscent of an infant, you don't start out running, you learn how to crawl, then walk, then run. Make a plan, know your limitations, and go follow it.

Notes: 5-on Graphs: Graphs in books of recovery for the recovering are not simple for one to impress on another—we do not need to do this in this book, nor do I want to. Plus, it takes too much valuable space, leave that for the scientist. Most graphs are negative in nature, or so I believe, rather than supportive to the recovering. In most cases with graphs in this area of study, the person doing the measuring takes them out of assumptions; one example might be, calling a slip a relapse to get a bigger or smaller account, number. If you have two years recovery time, consider yourself one of the lucky ones, that my friend is simple and truthful.

☼

The Lonely Child

✦

[Commentary-stories]

Do you greet [or did you greet] your children when they were home from school? Did you take them to church, or simply tell them to go [by themselves]? Where is the MOTHER? Did you know she is one of the most precious gifts God has given to mankind?

It is funny when I think about it, children in particular, society buys dogs, cats, fish and birds for their apartments, to keep them company, to feel loved; some buy horses. And all of this is fine, but too often it is apparent it is for taking the place, the love place for children.

My mother's love for my brother and I never stopped during our highs and lows throughout our lives, me being 55-years old today. During my recovering years, she never criticize me, maybe she didn't understand, but none the less, she did not belittle me, overlook me, I credit her for being more noble than I would be in such a case. I realize, and I think she did also, no one can be or do everything for the other person, but we can be there for them, she was for me.

The little girl, the little boy—they run, and run away fast, and when they do run, they look for replacements—if you are not available, usable for them as parents. They'll follow the damned, if they can see love linger in them.

Why do children get ill, sick? Ask them and see what they will say. I worked for a Free Standing duel-disorder Hospital some years back, very well known throughout the country. I worked in the children's ward, and yes, I asked them simple questions, and here is what they answered:

"I want my mother...I want my mother...I want my mother," endlessly. Some said, "Where is my dad, is he coming to see me, when, when, when is he coming?" I can go on and on, but you get the picture. They would rather sleep in puke than leave their mother, and/or father.

I have child development qualifications in my degrees, where I can work with children, I never wanted to use that part of my education, and was forced to when my supervisor reviewed all the candidates at the hospital for backgrounds. She said to me,

"Mr. Siluk, why did you not tell us of the developmental qualifications with children you have?"

I said, with a hesitant voice, "I'm not the person for that kind of position; I only got the educational background so I could understand things better."

Then she said, curiously, "Why do you think you do not qualify to work in that department?"

I knew they were shorthanded, and needed qualified people, but I just felt I was a disciplinarian, having 11-years in the Army, and was too rigid. But my answer to her was honest and I said, "Because they are little people, and all I want to do is hug them [love them], and I can't in there."

She looked at me and the only thing she said, and she said it solidly, "You can report to the department, you will be a Senior Counselor there, and if you do not, please do not come back to work, we'll send you your check."

Well, I did report to that department. And I did learn a lot in there about their needs, but love, and a sober family was the most pronounced need I witnessed. They all wanted to go home. They all would live in shit if only they could get back their mother.

So if you are gone, go back home and get those kids; return and put a smile on their faces. The drugs and the alcohol will not put smiles on anyone's face, not even yours.

☼

Another quick story: Recently my sister-in-law, returned to her family, in particular to her daughter after three years. The daughter, son and father were living at our place for a period of time, and the mother was 6000-miles away. The little girl was always pale, ill looking, never having a smile, unless force on her by appreciation for the little things she was given in life by others. She even asked me once to go get her mother for her, but I sadly told her I could not. Alcohol or drugs were not related to this case. But the point I'm getting at is, 'What caused that smile to reappear?' To be restored? You know what it was, the return of the mother. Love you learn at home, and take it out into the world with you when you leave; where there is no love only sadness, you will find a lonely child. The love that a child learns in the home today will be brought to others throughout the world tomorrow.

≈◊≈

PART TWO

The Story of:

A Woman in Pain

✦

[Revised]

Introduction

Note: Originally written in 1990, and previously [2002] went up for the Nimrod Literary Award; revised only in structure, 2001-2003;—originally published in the book, "Chasing the Sun."

This story is somewhat graphic. It entails the pain of a woman in an ongoing drama; I call it circular pain. A death occurs in the family. An illness takes place. Torment and fear run around in circles. We are talking now of a period of time in a woman's life, when—for the most part, she was successfully employed, yet disguised herself from those outside her family, which was in particular, just her children,—then continued to play the role of a solidly lower middle class happy family.

Gracefully she kept the secret [the bad one that is, by not seeking help], which was that her nurturing family as she pretended it to be;—was if anything, a household filled with silent nasty cries for help, vulgar at times, an empty joke of an existence, a pretence of agony, if you don't mind, for lack of a better term. But she faced it, turned it around, and took the best out of the worse. To get the full impact of the story, you must follow up on reading the Afterward.

The Story
A Woman in Pain
The Bed

The moment Judy took off her cloths she knew something was wrong. She never understood the reasons for such an alerted instinct, but she had it none the less;

maybe it was built over the years by need, unconsciously. Like an animal's instinct to survival—they know when death waits them; yes she was cautioned, every inch of her said to be so.

She paused at the head of the bed, standing naked except for her panties, over-looking her alcoholic husband slowly emerging from a light sleep, like the dead arising out of a coffin. The chair to her right held her blouse and skirt. She had been married to him for twenty-years, twenty-two years, close to half her life; ten of which belonged to a slow but progressive disease called alcoholism.

He looked up at her with an air of superiority, not unusual, not at all, a drunken dominance filled his countenance; it was an old expression, looking at her now, not new, old, old and getting older; a ten year old one, one could say, a daily look almost, a nightly look for sure, and getting much too familiar for her system to withstand, or so her stomach and her throat told her. She was always nervous it seemed these days. The closer she got to the house, the steps in the house, going to the bedroom, the door opening to the bedroom, her stomach muscles started cramping, her legs got wobbly, and she started to sweat profusely. A stutter came from her mouth, no real words, just, "aw awwwww aaaa...' as if she might need to say something, as if it was expected or her, as if her inner being was trying to force her to say, 'stop,' not quite knowing what to say, she said noth-ing, and thought, why should she say anything, it was a matter of not why any-more, but rather how to survive this night; she asked herself, but it would haunt her though: '...why did I come home?'.

She could smell the pours of his skin, they reeked, smelled, showed signs of a rotting body; they were drenched with alcohol, reeking like garbage after you open a bag of it up after a week. It was a death smell. The dark gloomy damp bar came out of his pours like osmoses. As she stood there, forced to smell him as long as she remained stationary; she could picture the bar, the people, and the life they all live in—a horrid life that was repeated day after day after day, never ending, always the same.

The bar, the common place for people to meet one may say, now-a-days, where one congregates, and dies slowly:—as if there was no other sanctuary, haven in town; is this all life has to offer? It was a question that went through her mind; it was one of the few practical ones she reiterated to assure herself, "I still had sensibility."

She didn't notice anything out of the ordinary, the drunken ordinary environ-ment she was standing in,—in the room his cloths were laying all about as usual, torn off of him; she noticed his shirt, a button was missing, funny she thought, how she caught that, but she had sewed so many of them back on, it was old business I suppose. She picked it up to place it over another chair and after that went back to her bed, standing—standing by it as she was before. She had moved about to see what he would say, to see how safe she was. He was staring at her, silent for the moment, as she stood against the bed,—trying to make a decision to just remain standing was hard, or should she run, hide, what? When she wanted to run, she couldn't, her legs would not obey; just like a minute ago, she really wanted to run, run and never stop running; she had just hoped he would not have woken up, but he did.

It came again, his solid fearsome stare, a wild evil look—as he braced half his torso up from the bed trying to focus in the dark, on his elbows, like a black cat in the middle of the night dodging car lights, he shook his head, as the arch-light from outside slightly blinded him through the window; it was a chilled fall night, and he kept the window open; she had learned most alcoholics do that for some odd reason, to cool their hot bodies down, or so they can get air in their saturated lungs. Whatever it was, it was heat going out the window, another expense. He wanted fear installed in her as usual. This wasn't a friendly smile he was now creating on his old looking, at one time youthful face [for he was merely in his early 40's];—almost a smirk appeared on his drooping face, not quite but almost; he wanted something else, it showed on his face, the demand would come soon, but how she wasn't totally sure, yet she knew it would not be pleasant.

He ordered her now to undress herself in front of him, as he stared.

[Fretfully—] she told herself, "This isn't the man I married 22-years ago," for the—*umpteenth time.* This one had a demon in him, a spirit of torment, he liked to see pain, he liked control, and he liked the stench of the lifeless. He made sounds resembling a dying boar, a dying dog, moaning for his lost soul; there was also a lustful groaning demon in him, this one, she knew would dominate her, it was just a matter of time, minutes, if not seconds; when was the issue, not where or how or if.

[Undecidedly with watchfulness] She entered in the bed almost automatically, knowing she had to sooner or later,—lifting up the covers, sheets and blankets, putting her leg and thigh down on the bed first, watching every eye movement of his, holding the covers with the left hand—holding her breath with her chest and stomach muscles—securing her right hand on the bed in case, just incase she had to run, or something, it was always that something, that bothered her. Then like a snake coming out of nowhere just appearing, his long muscular arm hurried to her hair, grabbing it, pulling harder and harder on it until she succumbed to its jerks, she now let go of her breath, it had started, no need to hold it anymore she told herself. Face first, she fell into the pillow. Her thinking was blurred for a minute. Mentally she was becoming stressed and drained, not unusual, not new just more bad memories 'on top of new ones,' she told herself, new ones to be; you never get used to it, never ever she told herself, no one does. You wait for it, know it going to happen, and when it does, again you ask, 'why, oh why,' does he do this, and why oh why did I let it happen, all questions, no answers, no answers ever come surface, none, none, none…and you forget the why's along the way, and go on with life. And you add to this, '…but not this again,' for he doesn't change much his mode or thought process, actually he becomes too predictable.

Then he pushed up his body, so he could see her, and peered over her like a rattle snake ready to devour a frog. Whatever he wanted he would take was written all over his face, with or without her consent, matter of fact, approval was never part of the equation in the past ten years. She was the scum of the earth right there, his whore, prostitute, the way he liked it, his bitch and his pussy, they were all words he liked to use, and he used them well, in the bed, at the bar, in the kitchen if he had a hangover, she knew in a minute he'd use them, and so part of the game was to anticipate, and be good at it. She told herself once if not a thousand times, this is not the love a woman needs, this is the way of a selfish man.

She closed her eyes, knowing whatever happened maybe, just maybe she could hide like an ostrich. Hide from this madman. A tear was hidden beneath her eyelid, just one; the dam, wall, barrier was not broken yet, although there were many cracks in it, she was the dame; he was the dame-breaker. 'He wants to see the tear again, just one, I know it, but I will not let him SSEEEE…' she told herself, in the form of a crying mumble. It would be his price, for peace, his prize to show and tell later while in a drunken stupor at the bar.

"What…tt did ya say whore…?" he muttered.

He shot a glance directly into her eyes now, as she opened them to see what his right hand was up to, she witnessed it was going onto her thigh,—then he started stroking it like a man ready to rape, like a man with sadistic-passion. But then she mumbled again,

"I've been raped a thousand times, once more, just more painful, another night." She told herself, it sounds the same, 1000 or 1001 times, or whatever, umpteen times. After the 1st time, the second, third, you get accustomed to it, she had in the past [for convenience sake] told herself, you just endure it the best you can. It seems normal after awhile, kind of normal, normal in a peculiar way, she told herself, questioning her own intelligence of what normal is and is not,— also, who is normal around her, and who is not. The next question, or thought was, 'why do I have to ask such silly questions on normality?' She knew when she had to ask that question, something was wrong, very wrong…possible sickly wrong or becoming sickly.

Like a thief in the night, he grabbed her groin area, and plucked out some hair. Then he did it a g a I n,

A N D

A

G

G ggggggggggA

IN

A N D A G A I N.

[Excruciatingly] The sound of her agony was seeping out of her body, as if it had its own internal expressions, idiom, for she was silent as far as she knew. Her body twitched here and there, automatic responses. You could hear the pulling of the hair in her crotch area, ripping of her hairs out, the stretching of her groin. It hurt, injured, and wounded her insides, her mental stability. She wiped the tears with the pillow. "He saw that one," she cried, "He likes seeing me cry," she said, but once he has seen it, his glory would be feed, victory would be his. It was a game for him. She didn't know why he liked it, but his face only got more excited when she did cry, an awful excitement, stimulation he had, as if he had won a jack-pot. On the other hand, she was in a dark anxiety, a world no one came to, no one wanted to come to, and surely, no place to be rescued from; a black hole filled her brain, she had now shut out everything and everybody, disassociation had taken over, she was, but she was not;—she was in a stalled state of existence [catatonic] and nightmarish in nature. As if she had stopped at a stop sign, and couldn't get the car back in gear, she was stuck for the moment. The dark shadows in her mind followed dark shadows circling her eyes, it wasn't, normal reality, but it was hers, and a way to endure.

She thought God made this human being: broad shoulders, strong, nice looking, and brown hair. He didn't make him to do such things like this to other human beings, to treat another person's body is such a brutal way, as if it was an abomination to mankind, to womanhood, God didn't make him to do this, he made himself to do this.

"I was a pretty woman at one time. People told me so. I was cute, they said, pretty, thin," she told herself, face smashed into the pillow.

She read his thoughts, after 22-years, one can do it pretty well.

He said,

"Don't say a word, don't wakeup the KID-Ssss. If you dare womaN, you'll be sorryyy." Yet he was a kid in his own way...the alcohol had stunt his growth. He was no more a man than a dead horse, or dog.

She remained silent, and used. His breath was a long lasting unendurable stink, reek, stench, as dry and stale as could be, beyond words...it never seemed dispersed properly, but circled around his bed, everlasting...why didn't it fly out the window she asked herself, everything else does, the heat, his bad language, but not the stink, not his bloody pores that reek booze; no, it's got to stick around and punish the co-dependent. She knew what she had become, even went to a support group once, a long time ago.

She tried to shift her face away from his; the putrid smell was noxious, deadly as he tried to stick his long lizard tongue in her mouth. It was full of white foam, white with saliva dripping,—saliva dripped upon her face, slobbering on her breasts, and neck. He bit her nipples, and covered them with her hands; her body shook at that event, shook and shook, he liked that, it was what he wanted, her thin body to move as if she wanted to make love. He gritted his teeth as if he wanted to bite them off. He was playing, but she wasn't. His breath was in the vein of toilet water. "God," she mumbled to herself, "This is the man I loved." She thought for a minute what she said, 'loved,' not love. She shook her head asking herself, "Who is he?" She again asked herself, and at that time out came the word "love, love. Oh, what kind of love

LOVE

L

O

V eeeeeeeeeeee is this?"

She knew now, beyond a doubt she did not love him, but loved him at one time, a time in the past. Yes they had a history together, but history is just that, the past, it is not the future. And that is what she was leaning toward. She cried repeatedly to herself as he shoved his whiskered face against her face, scratching it, as if it was wood on sandpaper. He liked it; she knew that. "He feels like a man's man now," she inarticulate cried softly into her pillow.

He now moved his body, positioning himself over her. She was all of 100-pounds; he was close to 200. Her panties were half ripped off by his rustic impulsive actions; not even knowing what he was doing he brushed her hips, by doing so. He took his off, ripping them with his knees, showing the barbaric, the caveman he was, and liking how he felt when he did it; and swearing all the way until he tucked them at the end of the bed under the covers with his feet, as if to say, out of sight, out of mind.

With a sigh, she whispered to herself, "NOW, he will want the sex, intercourse, fucking, not making love, just the F U C Kkkkkinggggg part, just sex, what a hero…why not fuck a hole in the wall, why me, why me…"

Having thought that, he pushed his body close to hers, and somehow, got her legs spread, the quest was on; they were tight, and her muscles were contracting like the contractions of a woman in labor. He put his hand on her pelvis as to secure it like a horse about to be ridden. Her legs and lower part of her body didn't want to obey his commands, they were resistant, they were trying to give him a message, as one does when the body is dying, but his body weight, and his powerful legs dominated hers, and she was subdued; oh yes, subdued like a cow being tied to be branded. As gasps of air came from her stomach, her eyes opened up as if to pop out. Now they were eye to eye, she had come out of her cocoon, what more could he do. Pressure was on her back, as her spine started going into spasms. Her whole body seemed to go into shock, disbelief, but not her mind, "Thank God," she said as she caught her breath—again, and being thankful for being conscious.

The gentleness that once came along with this act of husband and wife, making sexual love, was gone. There was no soul or feeling involved, no sensitivity, or sensuality; no warmness, or joy; no building up to a climatic euphoria, as heaven might say, 'heaven on earth'—none of this was present. The character of the soul was tarnished, and it was being poured out in hot venom onto her body. As she understood, love to be, she could not feel anymore; it was missing—just the fuck was present. The enjoyment of sex, what the preacher talked about at church was no more. His enjoyment was anger-pleasure, trying to get a high for relief, not happiness that is supposed to come with it. All he wanted was his dick sucked, like a Popsicle, and his way of thinking was, 'do it and be done with it,' no more, no less. She could remember the love making between them, it used to be 24-hours a day, that is to say, it was the little things throughout the day that made it so good at night: the touch, the hugging, the smell of his aftershave, and the smell of his skin, the fresh smell of his skin, his hair with nice curly waves of sweat luscious sensuality that came with her combing it with her fingers, and the warmth he gave over the phone, when he called her at work, and at times at home. She'd keep the phone to her face a moment longer after they had hung up; just caressing the warmth of his voice he left behind. It was all gone now. Like the bare apple tree in fall, all gone, a new season had come.

The Pain

"God," she said out loud, "please". He didn't hear anything, although she wasn't crying for help from him, she was just hurting and needed to hear herself; God was with her, she knew it, because the pain was too deep to endure for one person; the emotional roller coaster was on. He was over her now, and pumping her, fucking her like there was no tomorrow; in and out like she was a machine he drove his body. She didn't know why she accepted the endless hurt, maybe it was like the addict, or alcoholic, she never really understood, she was caught like a fly in a spider web. Where do you go with your life, it's here, or was it?

The pain filled her every pore, he wouldn't let up, and it was colored with shame, self-pity, worthlessness, agonizing adjectives, such as helplessness and unworthiness. And the physical was disjointing almost. Her bones shifted with his body. Sticking to his sweat, he pulled her up closer to him by her ass, squeezing it as if it was a teddy bear, until she groaned, and it was not a moan of pleasure, but rather one of dismay.

As he continued with his act of bliss, she thought: "…who would ever have me, now." And he pushed his weight, up and down, like a madman jacking off [masturbation], trying to hurry up and get to the end, the end, the best moment, the highlight of this affair, he was getting tired though; in addition, he wanted to get her attention, get her out of her dream spill, her thinking, he wanted her frightful attention. He wanted her to feel it, enjoy it, like him. But there was no way possible for that, she was numb from head to heal. His cock stuck inside of her akin to dogs. She was dry, and he was not merciful.

[Feeling destroyed] She said to herself: "…he's treating me like a cow, a piece of used meat, property, sucking on my breasts, as if trying to get milk from them. Slobbering, wet all over my torso. My legs, my arms, my stomach, my love area; I am no more than a commodity, like sugar. Who then would treat me with…C A R E, L O V E?

A P P R E C I A T I O N,

R E G A R D?

W

O

O

O ooo Ω….?

She allowed him to push harder on her pelvic bone; it seemed as if it was going to break. She dare not say a word, though. She had learned that the hard way: she was better off not coming home than say no. She had to wear dark glasses to work many of times when she said that forbidden word 'no'. He never remembered either that he hit her, pushed her around, fucked her hard, had no appreciation for her working and helping with the bills. He broke a few ribs when she defied him once; she remembered that well, he even told her, 'Can't you ever forget that." How one can forget, she'd mumble, when it never stops. But the black and blue eyes came more steadily. That was a fear of hers, loosing sight someday, getting damaged so bad she'd never be able to see, walk or talk again. This was not uncommon in her world, you simply needed to go to the bar and look at the other wives. He'd do something wicked, more wicked, more depraved, as time went on, and forget it, and say in the morning, "Gee, I don't remember, sorry."

Being sorry does no good, she knew this for a fact;—sorry was a word that was good for nothing, used by many people, but good for nothing. It was a cheap word for someone who was not responsible, one who liked their way, but not responsibility.

She said to herself, "I'm no more than a *horse, being ridden by a maniac…a half dead man. No more, any less. Just a quicken horse.*" Her mind was trying to keep up with the shock it was enduring. Reality would set in tomorrow morning.

"Can't…h…e…see what he's doing?" she cried as she stuck her head in the pillow again, hiding, trying to hide from the pain the shame. But instantly when she hid, he pulled her hair, it came out of her head; he now was looking at it. She was still in the pillow.

She was screaming inside "STOP, STOP…stop, no more!" But he continued, with a face that showed no mercy, no love. For all concerned, he could have smoked a cigarette doing the act, but he knew his dick would shrink, and he'd loose the pleasure, and then he would be mad as hell. She knew this to, and was hoping he'd pop before the cigarette entered his mind. "God Forbid," she thought, "if I have to stay up half the night sucking his dick to get it hard for a fuck he couldn't deal with. And on top of that go to work in the morning, all smiles."

She thought, and thought and thought, "If I was to be judged, let it be by God, not man," for she saw no pity from him, she wanted to kill him. At least get the damn hard-on, and get it over with. He had inserted his penis, but had a hard time maintaining an erection while inside of her, nothing new. But if you got to endure it, at least keep it hard she again mumbled.

"What did you say," he commented. She didn't answer, it was best not to. She pretended not to hear.

He was trying to hurry in fear he would loose it completely, now—the erection that is. He wanted his climax, his high, like his beer, quick and without reservation, or emotion. He was almost in a bear hug with her, trying to get that moment, the climax, afterward he'd fall to sleep, as usual. "The only difference between his liquor and me" she mumbled, "was the act." One took a hand to hold, as in a bottle, the other to shove his penis into my private part.

She prayed, and prayed, as he was going faster and faster, pushing his body in a chaotic way, "Don't slip, you'll rip me, please don't slip…" For sometimes he'd miss his aim, and his penis would come out, and upon inserting it again, miss again, and try to jam it in the wrong area, and she'd jump a mile. He thought it was because of his big penis, but it never got bigger than his thumb anymore, he was too drunk to keep the erection past a few minutes; plus all his energy went within the first five minutes, and it took him that long to figure out where to put it.

She thought, "I hope I do not have to guide the asshole so he wouldn't rip me like a hog again." He never knew the difference sometimes between what areas to enter. Thinking my asshole was the vagina.

He was in ecstasy now, and if it was not a pretense, he was the only one in ecstasy.

"Oh…o o o," he said in a drunken stopper. She was even more hurt now; the pain was in the core of the heart, knowing he was drawing pleasure from her hurt. He was climaxing. "Oh God," she cried, "Why, why does he do this to…to MMMMMeeeeee!" The tears were rolling over her cheekbones to her lips, salty, but pure tears.

She thought "He is shaking his head as if he is getting it off good. He even turned his head from me. He said '…indy', he's even thinking of someone else." Similar to a giraffe stretching his neck to reach a branch, he arched his body, his spine, back, to get the last ounce of cum from his internal organs out; after that he took a deep breath, and like a falling pillar, pushed once more, harder into her, until he sunk into his nest as far as he could go.

"Oh Lord, she sighed, "I'm so glad only you can see this."

He pulled his penis out as fast as he put it in. She was ripped from the roughness. She was now bleeding. Then like a rat gnawing on a piece of meat, he started plucking her groin area, again. He chuckled. She stared at him with fright, almost in a coma of shame; followed by him looking at her naked pitiful body, he said,

"You liked every minute of it bitch." She didn't respond. "How far from the truth can a person be," she thought. She endured it, despised it. Words could not describe her surface feelings, or her inner emotions. This was not a man thing to say, for she knew him when he was not a drunk, and was very careful in love making, it was a demon-possessed thing to say.

She moved from his sight, to her side of the bed. She was feeling, excruciating pain, emotional disarray, and physical soreness. He turned to his side as one would shut a car door and positioned himself to go to sleep. It was all of 12-minutes. The crisis was over. The man was an island, alone in a house full of love, with a family wanting him to heal, she thought. He speaks a different language though, different than the rest of us; he only understands his drunken world. It is his world, his demon made world.

"He can't love," she told herself. "Love is giving, he isn't capable; he loves the alcohol, for that is what he gives to. He is kinder to it than me," she thought, "He treats it better than me. Makes love to it, caresses the bottle. Not like me, who he treats like a horse, hog, and whore."

Thinking

[Disillusioned—laying along side her bed, her husband passed out.] Her inner self was analyzing the evening, the lost moment. "Hell," she said to her spirit deep within her mind, "He'll wakeup in the morning not remembering half of what he did—a black out—and I'll be left with the scars.

Even if I told people the way he was, what I had to put up with," she thought, "…they wouldn't believe me." And so she never did tell.

"In God's name why does he not stay at the bar, and not come back, back, back, here, stay gone," she cried. Adding, "I don't feel like I am a strong or a woman with courage, I feel simple, a survivor, and not so good at that either, tested under fire if anything."

"I would cry hardship, not sure if you get any more points from heaven for it. At 45-years old I have more wrinkles than an 80-year old woman. We all want heroes, I do, my hero was just a man of honor, I didn't even get that; he was no more honorable than I was happy.

He stays because I take care of him, take care of him. Put up with him. Is there no escape from this hell? Every time I walk in this room he's dead drunk, the walls whisper, 'trap, trap.' But I still come in." She tortured herself with rhetorical questions, question-statements, but where were the answers, she was not starting to ask for them, at least in her mind, in the corner of her brain, subconscious, they were surfacing, surfacing, surfacing, little by little.

As she looked over her shoulder, he moved like an uneasy and dying buffalo. Then she said in a low voice,

"Why do I go on like this, am I sicker than you?" The more she stared at him, that question flooded her brain. He was sleeping reminiscent of a bear in hibernation.

"Am I really sicker than him, **him him** him him mmmmmm." Then she questioned herself more, "I mean what person would allow such behavior to be put upon them? Sick, sick, sick, I'm sick Sick, SICK,…S I C K."

As she pulled the covers over her body, she curled up into a shell, like a worm;—a closed form, like a fetus trying to keep warm in her mother's womb, approximating, a turtle trying to hide in a shell. She didn't want to share her thoughts, not even with God for the moment. Her pain was humiliating, very deep humiliation, shame, SHAME.

As she tossed and turned with the covers and pillow, she started talking to herself, "I have always got paid for my duties, like at work," she said in a mumbling voice, "And I don't have to accept this kind of physical and emotional abuse, but why do I?" 'Don't have to keep…' continued to emerge in her mind: don't have to, don't have to…

[The dilemma started to crack] She hesitated with open eyes, looking out from her bed into the dark room. Shadows from the cars passing by hitting the streetlights reflections, bouncing through the shades of her window: she whisperers to herself, knowing he now is heavily asleep, and he got his morbid pleasures, no reason for him to wake up, she whispers,

"The shadows are more comfort than this dead drunk body lying next to me." Then says, while talking to herself '…it's ok to talk to yourself, who else can I talk to?' She speaks to God:

"An ark light on outside, leave it on, God leave it on. So I am not alone with this beast. The shadows are my company; a silent world for the most part, even heaven is silent." But the shadows and the horns, and the sound of car tires kept her mind busy, away from his dirty deeds that have been done to her, that in itself is god sent.

[Restlessness] "You're saying something," said her husband, tossing and turning, trying to get into a comfortable position to sleep. Insomnia had crept into his life the past couple of years; if booze couldn't put him to sleep, which it did often times, but he would always wake up sporadically throughout the night, yet, it didn't resolve his sleeping needs, it actually deprived him. She continued to talk to herself, knowing he was talking in his sleep,

"He used me as a fuck tool to get him to sleep. He screwed me until he got exhausted, and then fall to sleep," the bastard. She was angry, twitchy but something else was happening…at the same time, she was becoming motivated, aggravated to the point of being hungry for release, release with freedom; freedom to be hungry for life. It was either, stick with the hunger for freedom, or die being beat to death, or third option, join the drunken lifestyle of his and not give a shit. But the hunger for freedom was weighing heavy. She didn't quite know what came along with freedom, but it left him out of the picture.

"I hate who he's become," confirmed Judy, as the night got older. "The damn alcohol was no true lover. It steals, robs, and kills you, slowly, similar to boiling a person alive. It takes your money, your family, your sleep, your hunger, and yet he wants more. It's insane. And I'm insane for being part of this conspiracy."

This man was a professional drunk, not an amateur she was learning. He knew when to use it, make her feel guilty, a form of anger-control, and he had mastered it.

The booze had kept him busy, and had saturated his whole damn life—

—this she was now piecing together; she had time now, the night was dark, good for thinking, he was out, solidly out, and the sounds of the chilled streets set the perfect atmosphere for thinking, deducing, and analyzing, and conceptualizing.

It was sleep he needed for the moment, a fuck a few minutes ago, drinking a few hours ago, yesterday his family, he will want his family to gush over him at breakfast—as usual, and his heart—which was weak, will get weaker. What would be next in his life? Better yet, as she stared out the window, the question came: 'what next in her life…?' [She deduced his was over.] For ten years it was all for one, not any other combination, such as, 'one for all and all for one.'

[Exhaustedly] She asked herself, "I wonder why, why doesn't he know he will die from this crap? I suppose he does someplace in that black out unconscious mind of his. He must," she questioned herself.

His gastrula system was that of a man who lost his automatic control valves. It was out of control. He farted until he almost shit in his pants, and many times he'd wake up walking with shit hanging from the hairs on his ass, trying to get to the toilet in time, as it ran down his legs. Disgusting as it was, it was also pitiful to witness, Judy had told herself, and as he sat on the toilet, she'd clean it up.

"Why not him, why does he not clean his own shitty tracks up, why not…?" a good question [a question never asked, or answered] that was now seeping out of her mouth as she stood next to the window, looking at the cars drive by. "Wh…y…Nooott?" she repeated herself. After that, as a loud truck drove by, she answered her first question, "I don't know why not, but I should!" That was the same answer he gave her when she'd ask him, 'Why don't you stop drinking,' he'd say 'what for [forgetting the 'why not'],' and drink another beer. "Funny, funny," she told herself, until the evening seemed to close in even closer to the point of no return.

[Talking out loud now to herself] "He transforms into the demon, you know, sometimes he shits full packs into his pants when he gets into bed, not even taking off his cloths; lumps of shit in them. That's when I sleep downstairs on the sofa. His farts are long, as long and loud as those damn Wednesday 1:00 PM, alert horns the city blows, testing for an emergency; here right here is an emergency. Two or three minutes I think, yes, two or three minutes for the fog horn and the farts to end. I can endure them, but the lumps of shit, no way."

His eyes would be red in the morning, his skin a pal green, sickly, liken to the pale rider in Billy Graham's books on the four horsemen, she told herself. That is what he looked like, like death. His short-term memory was shot as hell, a man at 45, or was it 46 now, she had to guess, her memory was going also, "I can't remember it…his damn age." She had now calmed down, her body had stopped racing. He wouldn't remember tomorrow what he did, matter of fact, he wouldn't remember—if he was sober at this moment—two hours earlier," she spoke with reprisal, yet what was coming to mind was not vengeance in the sense of aggression, but rather of freedom. That was the best revenge she could give. Simply move on, and forgive him, so she could live.

"For god's sake man stop your farting and go to hell," she thought as he turned back to his position again in the bed trying to get a pillow under his stomach. She was just about to ask the rhetorical question, the one people go to hell for, "When are you going to die?" "Oh God," she thought, "Did I think that?" Was I going to say that, "When are you going to die, and go to hell?" She heard a voice in her head, 'yes, you already said it'," God for give me." She cried, "Yaw, I did" She told herself. "I sure did. I said it in my mind, and out loud. Almost spit it out." She added, "I don't want him to go to hell, I just don't want to live in his hell; nor do I want him to die, but he is going to die anyways."

Her mind went shifting into a vortex of images like a ship in a storm; the sounds of the cars seem to have a language of its own, a calming sound. Only she could understand it though, like a rhythm; then it was quiet. And then the sound of rain hit the car wheels, but it wasn't raining, it just sounded like it for some reason.

◇

"I've taken care of three kids, and...and...a...child adult. I go, go...o to work everyday, while he sits at home and ponders on jealous thoughts to confront me with...why, what have I done to deserve this. Do I not have a perfect track record, I've never cheated on him,—every evening without missing one I come home, wait for him, or meet him at the bar, unless he is sleeping, dead to the world, then I stay home and wait for him to wake up? Evenings are for the devils." She told herself, "Not for me. I live in a home that I dread coming home to. I hate evening."

[Insightfully dreary, she now lays back into her bed] "Is every alcoholic that damn jealous," she mutters out the side of her mouth, thinking she was going to get an answer, but none comes. She could hear herself talk, she could hear her voice, the car tires, see the shadows in the room. She could read his mind also. He wanted to punish her for his misery.

She had heard that alcoholics get jealous, that it was a characteristic of theirs, and seeing believed, and it was true, very true. And now she was part of the roller coaster, and believed it, believed it because she was living it. They say love is being kind, caring and all such things, that again is what she was brought up to believe. But there was no kindness in this house.

And so she framed in her mind what the drunk shows love to be, and it was jealousy, yes, love is jealousy to the drunk, love is paranoia full time, impurity part time. Her husband was sleeping proof of this analysis.

He never feels safe, she told herself, always editing himself, like a man who really had something to hide. "The only thing he had to hide was his shit ass treatment to me, and hides from everyone else. Saying to me, 'no one needs to know our business,' as if it was a business, treating me as crust off a dirty stove. And I helped him with that." Furthermore, she went on to say, while talking to herself in bed, pushing the pillow here and there, a trait of her husband's restlessness, "It is the family thing he'd say, 'keeeeeeeppppp it in the fffamily, nOOO ones else's business.' That was the motto, a stinking cover-up motto."

[Consoling herself] 'Hell,'" she said to her inner soul, "I've been faithful beyond reason," thinking why not have an affair?—Which was picking up in the corner of her mind,—it was justified, alright. "Who would blame me? Why not have one, he has. Give me a good reason not to have one," She questioned her mind; no answer came. Talking to herself again, she pointed to the many women he knew, at the bar, here and there, everyplace he'd, or they'd go. And the many men he knew that would come on to her when he wasn't looking.

"They'd like to grab my ass; no they did grab my ass; and not as hard as he did. He'd say nothing, or imply, they were just joking around. If I'd say nothing, he'd kick my ass in the morning saying, I let them and I like it, you can't win."

But she couldn't she convinced herself, it wasn't her; that was him, to take another drunk on, would be simply stepping from one garbage can to another. "It was really beyond reason," she continued to tell herself. "To get better, to save the mind, you can't duplicate bad behavior she convinced herself. Plus, I have values, if I go against them, I could never live with myself. A drunk no longer has them, no values, and no feelings of bad behavior, when they violate them; they have no character in their soul left." She told herself.

Although, thinking she had good reason to have an affair, but couldn't, she put that thought to rest. She knew every time this happened these thoughts surfaced, would go through her head, never did anything about them, just thought them. Like his jealousy, after she came back home from wherever he was, he'd get his anger out, and the jealousy would subside a few hours into the night. Having an affair was hard she concluded each time this idea emerged, anyone of his so called good-friends would jump in bed when he wasn't looking in a minute, it just surfaced, and then sank back into where it came from, some quicksand someplace hidden in her brain. And in most cases, who would know she had an affair anyways? if she had one.

"The bar, the bar the bar, that's all they think about. Let's meet at the bar. I'll see yaw at the bar. The bar is home, the fucken bar robs you, but no one said that." She whispered to the shadows, to the sound of the cars, tossing and turning in bed.

He mumbled out loud again, something unutterable; as he started to hurl and rotate his dying body like a worm trying to cross the street before it's baked alive. His heavy breathing started, it was noticeable, as if his heart was not pumping right, as if it was overworking, compensating for his messed up whole biological system. His heart was weak, and getting weaker as years went by. He had had two heart attacks previously, and he was 46, just forty-six. She said to the shadows, that looked like eyebrows on the bedroom ceiling, as if they would notice her seriousness, she said, as she turned to look at him, glancing away from the window, and shadows, and knocking out the sounds of the cars, she said with a tear in her eye,

"You're killing us all, you're drinking, you're having, and wanting to have power over everything, your madness, your jealousy, and envy's...everything is like a sick cow. That is what it is, a sick...sick...cow. And your self-pity, like a man running away from the draft, a coward and a sick, sick coward-cow. Life is robbing you—you and you and me and me, and you don't even know it, sick, sick cow. But I...I...I...I...III know it."

She cried but a few more tears, holding in a hurricane, a rainfall-of-tears,— lying on the bed, her chest trying to recover from the thinking, she closed her eyes.

≈

[Sleepy] "And I'm sure it was my fault," she continued to tell herself; "...that is what he would say at least."

Next she thought about the times they would meet his friends at the bar, and he'd laugh with his friends, not with me she thought. "He gave me the shitty attitude with them. I was his buffer, safeguard, also his sacrifice, and his fucken cow to milk when he wanted. Grab a little ass when he wanted to show off.

He drank like he fucked me, like a man ready to be put in an electric chair, as if it was his last meal. I owed him. Society owed him." She thought, "Everybody owes him."

Tears rolled from her dark brown closed eyes, salty full tears, rolled over her checks, down around her lips, and on to her neck, across her light complexion they continued until the tears healed her wound. She had learned not to show her weakness, he would only play with it, if not use it against her. She told herself many times, "Don't let him find my weakness he will use it against me," plus, she'd add, "I'd be left with no, not one, no not any, defense." That is how he thought, she contrived, how he played the game. But he was the only one allowed to play. She opened her eyes and looked at the clock; it was tomorrow now, a new day. And so she added with a smile, her first smile after such an ordeal, "The game should have two players, not one." Having said that, she took a deep, deep breath and closed her eyes again.

☼

[Amazingly, with new strength] She had come to the conclusion, it wouldn't help for her to tell anyone at work, if she did, they would simply say *don't bring your problems to work*; or would it help to tell her family, no, they would only scold her for accepting it; some more humiliation, dishonor, shame. But she had to do something, something quick, while she had this new found strength. Things come and go, especially emotions, and then the thoughts are tucked away for another day, and so she knew it was *'act now or never.'*

"If I run out of the house, it would be like old times. I run to a shelter, a police station. The children and I sit and wait, and wait. By morning time, I got to go to work, put the kids in school; he gets a good night sleep. I get the chair in the Police Station with three kids. I get to the shelter, he shows up. Police come. I talk to him, he is sorry, I go back, and everything is fine, although I did put him in jail once. But I will never do it again. My kids, his family, my family, everybody chose him; I went too far they all said. He ended up being the damn hero. Unbelievable; but things change, or so they shall."

The Secret

[The next day] She put up a shield, screen,—told to her loved ones and friends not a thing about her life, or her husband's lifestyle. To all that observed, her household was as it was portrayed, quiet and serine. And the few times it got out of control, chaos, it would pass.

But the truth of the matter was that it was not so serine ever, and nothing ever functioned right. And if it ever did for a moment in their lives it was because Judy cultivated it, and aged before her time.

It was morning now. As he sat at the kitchen table he grabbed the paper from the counter thumbing through the first few pages to the sports, looking at Judy with a smile. Then it was that a strange thing happened. She thought [mustering up some hidden courage, she came up with the idea the end of the world was not here, not today, she had a choice] "...goddamn, he had a blackout again; he doesn't even remember a thing, does he?" She was crying with bittersweet tears inside, deep down in her core, tightening up her jaw, teeth on teeth. A tear crept from her eye, but somehow, out of pure will, she stopped the rest of the tears from coming up to flood her face, and reminded herself of the belittlement, torment, shame, disregard he thrust [and sanctified] upon her the night before. But not a spoken word was uttered between both of them during the first few minutes of contact.

He leaned back in his chair, coffee hot in front of him, like a king, dirty shirt, messed up hair, as if he had a bad housekeeper, as if he had a lazy wife, or so these thoughts went through Judy's head.

Another tear surfaced, it had a long way to get to her eyes, but it did, and she couldn't stop it. Her will was not strong enough anymore. She turned around so he wouldn't see it, rubbing her eyes as if they were sore. He smiled, as if to say, in a dumbfounded way, anything wrong, but chose instead to say,

"Make me some eggs honey."

[Cringing] She knew not what to say, she knew what she wanted to say though, 'no', for that is what she wanted to say, but say it loud, "NO, NO, not until you read my hurt," but she didn't say it. Just not having him remember the drunken stupor he had, the awful treatment he put her through, was painful for her…"Remember, remember asshole," she told herself, but not him. Everything was silent, he knew something was wrong.

[Dizzy with stressful thoughts] "The dirty, slobbering fucken love making you shamed me with last night, is what this silence is all about, forced sex, forced shame, trying to rape my soul, make my soul red like yours."

That is what was going on within the tight stern face she couldn't get rid of, the tired hate in her eyes. The sound of her mind ticking away the minutes and seconds, for soon she would be walking out that door, to go to work and get renewed.

"Honey…" he said with a thought on his mind.

She didn't turn around from the stove, her back was to him, she thought, "…your honey is in the damn bottle, have it make your eggs, why am I standing here making your eggs?" But she started to pull out the egg pan, thinking, he never relies on himself to do anything.

[Restiveness] That restlessness she was feeling last night, the insightfulness she felt was surfacing, surfacing…slowly, and the tears had come and gone, she was wounded, but the cut was healing.

The past ten-years, since he lost his job, Judy thought, as she prepared to make the eggs, he's really done nothing except, drink, make fun of me and the kids [the three children now were all over 18-years old, but all living at home.]; nothing at all to do but feel sorry for himself, while I bring home the check. And he wonders why he has a weak heart.

"Make the house payment that is what he cares about, NOTHING else, N O T H I N G…ING…more." She scolded herself mentally, within the corner of her mind, silently.

She knew, and had calculated that recently his physical abuse had worsened. "What's the future hold?" She thought. "He laughs at the idea that he may even have a problem with alcohol. He's 47…no 46, just 46, that's all, I forgot his age, yaw, 46, when is he going to grow up? Become a man? Be responsible? [Her back still turned away from him] He knows and I know he is a stinking ship, a drunk, a fucken Peter Pan toy."

She was always taught the two go together. That is, being a man, and being responsible. He just rearranged the life code of man, that's all. And would arrange for her to do whatever needed to be done, and that included her life code. "Where was his strength, in his damn penis," She thought "in his mouth, his fists?"

"These eggs will never get done," she mumbled.

"What was that honey," He responded.

"Oh nothing, just talking to myself, these eggs seem to take forever."

"Yaw, honey, just don't worry, take your time," he said as he kept reading the paper, occasionally look above the paper to see if she was cross with him, not remembering much of the night before.

As she turned the eggs over to let them harden a bit, she asked herself: "…[Trying to clear her throat] he's always making me feel guilty; he's a master at it." But she remembered from that person at the support group, the one she went to just one time, that, alcoholics were good at survival, they used people to get to the next day. Promise the moon, and give a rock. They know how to make you believe what they want you to believe."

Unconsciously, she knew she was becoming more ill than him. Why else would she stay in a situation like this? Oh for many reasons. One being she was ill. Ill people stay with their kind, she had noticed from the past, and well people avoid them, so they do not get ill, maybe it's contagious. She asked her inner being.

But she needed love, love that gave, not love that took like a vampire, drawing all the blood and strength out of a person until there wasn't any left. She needed love that was not maladaptive; love that makes you see red, rather than black and blue, genuine love. It is what a woman needs, love and appreciation, and touch she told her heart. Not fucking out of anger, hate, scorn, and turning eggs over.

She was furious inside now. She needed to see a man's tear, his if possible. Any man would do. She had almost lost all her self-respect, self worth because of a man. "Do men cry?" She questioned herself. "I want to see," she hesitated, said a pray. "Please God," she asked, "Show me one tear by a man. Show me [she cried] a man in the human race, in man's kingdom, a man tear, anyone out there with a man tear!!

    A
      MAN
        T
         E
      A R R R R!!!!

Are not all men alike? It can't be so. 'No…No…'" she told herself.

Work & Breakfast

[With hope and resentment] As she readied herself, putting on her hat, jacket, picking up her purse, insuring her lipstick was on right. Wiping her eyes to insure her make-up was not smeared from the tears, and putting on a new morning smile, she walked out of the doorway, of the kitchen. Breakfast had been made, she had to go to work, she remembered the night before, how painful it was to endure, the insults, the slobbering, the passing out, after he had his kicks. How she was left used and alone, sleeping next to an island that needed only his next fix, drink, and fuck-something to satisfy his craving. He didn't care what form it came in, as long as it came. This was their life, what else she knew, she told herself.

[Slyly] She turned about looking at him, as he gave a big smile, giving her a wink, holding the paper in one hand, putting the coffee cup to his mouth, his eyes catching hers. She stared for a minute downward, it was not out of shame, but out of emotions she looked down, trying to release all the emotions caught inside of her. Then looking up thinking on the way up, she said, "Good-by, honey," she had never called him honey before, nor said goodbye in quite the same manner. It was his style she had robbed for the moment, duplicated if you will. He sat holding the paper and coffee, not drinking it, a frown came upon his face, not sure what to say.

As she started the car, she said to herself out loud, "I need more, much more. I need friends, dignity, and a renewed self. I need love that my husband sitting at the damn table eating his eggs, can't give. Even the sound of him slurping his coffee is starting to infuriate me. The one that says 'Honey', and later on in the evening when I come home, or he comes home, pisses his pants, the honey will be gone. I don't want his mess. I don't want to fuck him either, or sleep with him, he does not sleep, he passes out, dies a little each night. I would be more comfortable on the floor sleeping, and if that is where I end up so be it. I'll learn how to live," She told herself, "How to deal with a new life. If I can adjust to this kind, I can adjust to anything. I just have to find out what is normal again. I forgot." As she looked up at her living room window, she noticed he was standing there waving her goodbye, holding the curtain. He had taken the time to actually get up and walk to the living room, she said out loud in the car, "I can't believe it. He even left his paper and coffee in the kitchen." He waved again, but she never waved back. And she drove off.

Afterword

There is more truth to this story than fiction. For the sake of the story, let's say the husband died two years after that happened. And the lady did go to work that day. It was troublesome to say the least, only because she had to make a decision, that being, if she was going back into that house or not. She did not go back. She gathered her children and stayed with a friend. No fresh cloths for a week, not much money, and at the mercy of her friends, and having to tell the whole truth, and nothing but the truth.

Now let's say, she needed to get it out, her abuse, share it. Make it real. Make it public. When it wasn't' public, she had no chance of help. She learned that if it is a secret, then it should be a good one not a bad one. I am sorry about using the F word so much in this story, but it is in place I do believe, the non-fiction part demands it. Otherwise, normally I would not use the word.

Now again, let's put a nice ending to this story, he did die sober. He did go get help, and she did allow him to move back into the house after several months of sobriety. And no, he couldn't work again. But he was a better man. Not the same one who she married, but then she was not the same either.

It took her another two years to date, after his death, to build up strength. After that she met her first date; fell head over heals with him, which is not unusual in such cases. I think because he showed her respect it was easy for her to pick up a fairytale romance, not because they loved, and they may have, but because it was what was missing before. And possible the reason it didn't' work out for them, was, she couldn't tell the difference. But none the less, she went on to heal from that relationship to a more positive one. And yes, I would like to end this story by saying she is living happily ever after. And so there is hope out there. You don't change partners because you want to, it is not a good reason, you change because it doesn't and isn't going to work. Otherwise all you are doing is going from one person with baggage to another. We all have baggage you know. But let's hope before we start a relationship, ours has been taken care of, at least for the most part.

About the Author's Books

Tales of the Tiamat: This is a trilogy, consisting of "The Tiamat, Mother of Demon," the second book, "Gwyllion, Daughter of the Tiamat," and the third, "Revenge of the Tiamat". All three are full of adventures and travels by Sinned, the main character of the three novels, as is the Tiamat involved, yet we see many other antagonists along side of her. The series takes you to Malta, Easter Island, ancient England, and Avalon, where the Tor is being built, Asia Minor, where Yort is, Sinned's home, and a half dozen other places. In addition to the main story of each of these three books, which is being put into one, in the "Tales of the Tiamat," a fourth book was added, called "The Tiamat and the King," on which is the "Short book," added into the series, it is really the conclusion to the trilogy never put into the book. It was, for the most part, written during the same period of time the three were, and revised recently. It will be put into both the "Tales of the Tiamat," if this book ever comes out, and has been put into the book, "Death by Desire," again, if that book is ever published.

The Chick Evens Sketches: In this trilogy, we have sketches of life that incorporate the late 60's to the early 70's; the hippie generation, the new era, the awakening of Aquarius, the peace era, it has been called many things. In his first book, his sketches, take you on a romance of a city and era, the book being called: "Romancing San Francisco" [1968-69], he introduces us to karate's famous Yamaguchi family, to include Gosei, and his father Gogen "The Cat"; along with the famous Adolph Shuman, the once owner of the line of Lilli Ann cloths, along with other sketches. In the other two books, "A Romance in Augsburg," and "Where the Birds don't Sing," the sketches start where the first book left off, from 1969 to 1970 and to Vietnam in 1971. Here you go to Europe for a Romance with a Jewish German girl, and on to Vietnam where there is a war going on. Mr. Evens will also end up in Sydney, for one week of some great adventures, what the Army called back then R&R; Mr. Siluk spent 11-years in the Army, being a Staff Sergeant when he was discharged, and has lived all three books.

Short Story Collection [s]: this is not a trilogy, rather three books, of which two are similar, that being of Suspense, "Death on Demand," of which there are seven stories, and *"Death by Desire"* having ten; and the third book, being a mixture of short stories, called *"Everyday's an Adventure"*.

Spiritual: The Author has some strong religious and spiritual views. Having studied and done graduate work in theology, and missionary work in the mountains of Haiti, and being at an earlier age an Ordained Minister, his two books, *"The Last Trumpet and the Woodbridge Demon,"* being his first book in this genre, talks about experiences of the early eighties, where he had visions concerning end time events that are coming to pass right this very moment. In his second book, *"Islam, In Search of Satan's Rib,"* he talks about the ongoing subject of terrorism on America, and the world as a whole, but in a different manner; instead of trying to figure out the mind of the Islamic-Arab, he looks at this god, enmeshed with Islam today.

Addiction: As of this writing [August, 2003], Mr. Siluk is still a licensed Counselor in good standing with the State of Minnesota. He has also held international licenses in Drug's and Alcohol, and has worked for hospitals and clinics in dual disorder facilities. In his book, *"A Path to Sobriety, the Inside Passage,"* which is a common sense book on understanding alcoholism and addiction, the book is an ultimate guide to substance abuse, a powerhouse for preventing relapse and curing the disease. The book you are now holding in your hands called *"Prevention..."* is his follow up book [companion] to his *"Path to Sobriety..."* on addictions. Which he was not going to release depending on the need for it; but after the death of his mother, who helped him during his early stages of recovery, has chosen to finish it, and now release it. As in everything in life, school, the Army, training etc, you need a book to learn from, and one to practice with. This is the practice book, the hands on book you might call it, *"A Path to Relapse Prevention."* He is also, half way done with a book on *"Aftercare..."* which if published, would be his final book in the Chemical Dependency area, and series.

Travels: Mr. Siluk has travel, or has been traveling I should say for some 37-years out of his 55 ½ years of his life to this date. He has traveled 24 ½ times around the world. And in most of his books you can see, and feel and almost taste this [to be more exact, he has 613,000-air miles, not to include ground miles]. In his book, *"Chasing the Sun,"* he takes you to a variety of places, by showing you some forty-pictures,—giving you an overall view of his story on how he got started. Each picture has its own caption, and is read for 'a want to be traveler', or one who would like to reminisce.

The Beast Books: I wasn't sure what to call these three next separated books, so I named them, the *"The Beast Books"*. For in their own way, they all have their own beast. The first book being, *"Mantic ore: Day of the Beasts,"* which is the author's favorite of the *three, you step into the demonic underworld. A lot of him is in this book it seems. A touch of Vietnam, a touch of his home town, St. Paul, Minnesota, and the invisible shadows that change shapes into animals and human forms; visions upon visions. In the second book, the "The Rape of Angelina of Glastonbury, 1199 AD," which is also in a revised version, in the book "Death by Demand," you are involved with a suspenseful story of revenge, and at the end of the book is a nice surprise, another story. And for the third beastly book, "Angelic renegades & Rephaim Giants," you get just that, no more, no less. It is a book on the ancient dictators of the world, the ones who have cursed God, to have man worship them; for the most part is it sketches, impressions, and glimpses of this world.*

<u>*Out of Print book:*</u> *For the curious reader; although they are out of print, the author has a few left in storage. "The Other Door," was his first book published, in 1981, a book on poetry. It is a Volume one, of which he is working on volume two, yes, 22-years in the making. This book is so scarce that only 25-copies are left, at a price you most likely you would not want to pay. Second, is the authors 2nd book, "The Tale of: Willie the Humpback Whale," which got much attention in the year, 1982, although it did not get a Pulitzer Prize, it was an entry, and considered. At present the author is considering a 4th printing, and revised edition. He does have a number of copies available for interested people [a limited number]. And the book "Two Modern Short Stories of Immigrant Life," that is more of a chap book that came out in 1984 as a trial run. Only 100-copies were ever printed, of which one of the stories were printed in the, "Little People's Press," and then the book was pulled back for personal reasons, and off the market by the author. This very limited book of which there are possible 30-copies left can also be acquired, but again, this overview is more for the inquisitive than for selling these very rare and hard to find books.*

Visit my web site: <u>http://dennissiluk.tripod.com</u>

You can also order the books directly by/on: <u>www.amazon.com</u> <u>www.bn.com</u> along with any of your notable book dealers

Note: Picture on the back of the book is of the author, 1999, while in a boat off the coast of Iceland, spotting whales

0-595-29391-3